Registry Review in Computed Tomography

Registry Review in Computed Tomography

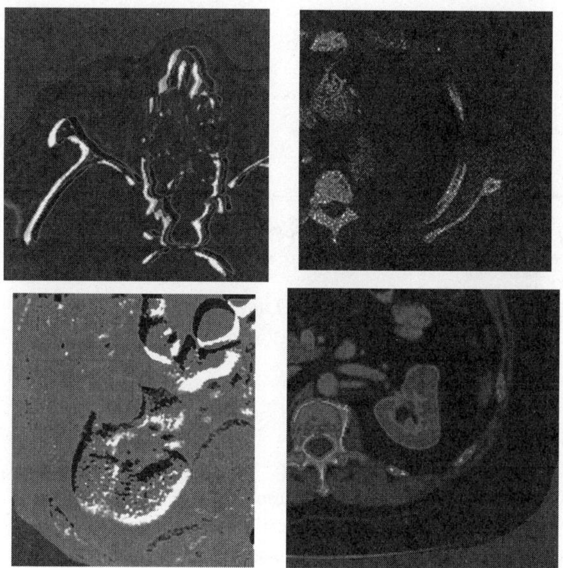

Daniel N. DeMaio, B.S., R.T. (R)(CT)
Assistant Director/Clinical Coordinator
Radiologic Technology Program
Long Island University—C.W. Post Campus
Brookville, New York

W.B. SAUNDERS COMPANY
A Division of Harcourt Brace & Company
Philadelphia London Toronto Montreal Sydney Tokyo

W.B. SAUNDERS COMPANY
A Division of Harcourt Brace & Company

The Curtis Center
Independence Square West
Philadelphia, Pennsylvania 19106

Library of Congress Cataloging-in-Publication Data

DeMaio, Daniel N.
Registry review in computed tomography / Daniel N. DeMaio.—1st ed.

p. cm.

Includes bibliographical references.
ISBN 0-7216-6285-4

1. Tomography—Examinations, questions, etc. I. Title.
RC78.7.T6D45 1996 616.07′572′076—dc20 95-49210

Registry Review in Computed Tomography ISBN 0-7216-6285-4

Printed in the United States of America.

Last digit is the print number: 9 8 7 6 5 4 3 2 1

For my parents, Robert and Emily

Preface

The American Registry of Radiologic Technologists (ARRT) has been instrumental in the advancement of diagnostic radiographers, radiation therapists, and nuclear medicine technologists since its inception in 1922. Most recently, the ARRT has attempted to further improve and promote the medical imaging profession and prevent professional obsolescence by including a continuing education requirement in its recertification procedure. As of January 1, 1995, technologists who wish to remain certified in their respective modalities by the ARRT are required to show evidence of continuing education.*

The mere mention of continuing education is enough to instill panic in many technologists. However, the idea of remaining informed of new developments and reviewing basic principles through continued learning is not a new one to many members of the health care system. The situation faced by radiologic technologists today is similar to that faced by nurses, physician's assistants, and physical therapists, among others. To many health care professionals these advances appear to be so overwhelming that it seems impossible to keep up.

However, continuing education can be a tool for self-improvement and cognitive advancement, not simply a forced responsibility or costly nuisance. First, many of the basic introductory principles one learned as a student may now be difficult to fully recall. Second, technology is advancing more and more each day. The next time you are at your

---

* Where applicable, please contact your state agency regarding continuing education requirements for maintaining licensure.

place of employment, stop for a moment and carefully examine your surroundings. How much have things changed since you were hired? Each day you rely on extremely complicated and sophisticated devices to complete medical imaging procedures. Do you completely understand how each of these devices operates? Many of our peers would say that it is not necessary to understand how each device works to become an effective technologist. Hopefully, a large majority of us disagrees. We know the importance of this fundamental information and also realize that any position in health care is tremendously more rewarding if you take the time to appreciate and truly understand the science and technology that surrounds you. This is certainly no easy task. The fact that there is continuously more to learn about our profession should serve as a great challenge to all of us.

When viewed with the proper perspective, continuing education can be seen as a path toward increased technical knowledge and professional advancement. It is also a much-needed method of retaining the respect of the public and our peers within the health care system. Remaining current within a field whose technology is rapidly changing can be extremely difficult. The ARRT requirement for continuing education is indeed a positive step. However, each of us must share the responsibility of remaining competent. It is a responsibility we owe to our patients, our coworkers, and most importantly, ourselves.

The ARRT has mandated as a continuing education requirement that every 2 years, all radiologic technologists must complete 24 hours of continuing education or must pass either an advanced-level examination or an entry-level examination that the technologist is eligible for. Confirmation of the fulfillment of this requirement is made by the technologist on the renewal form for ARRT certification during his or her birth month each biennium.

Continuing education courses can be found at local health care facilities, at colleges, and through private educational corporations. Entry-level and advanced-level examinations are offered by the ARRT three times each year. ARRT entry-level exams include those in Diagnostic Radiography, Nuclear Medicine Technology, and Radiation Therapy Technology. The ARRT continues to develop advanced-level examinations in addition to those currently available, which include Cardiovascular-Interventional Technology, Mammography, Magnetic Resonance Imaging, and Computed Tomography.*

Those of you who are reading these pages are undoubtedly eager to successfully complete the ARRT advanced-level examination in Computed Tomography. It is on this endeavor that we now focus our attention.

---

* Contact the American Registry of Radiologic Technologists for additional information.

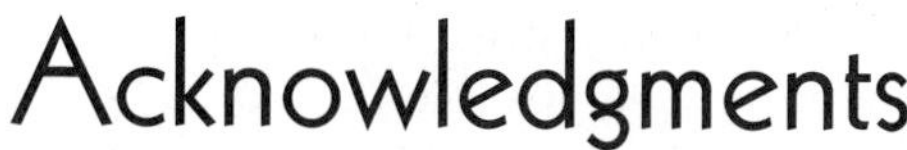

Acknowledgments

I wish to thank the professional staff of the W.B. Saunders Company for their help during the publication of this book. A special note of thanks goes to Ms. Lisa A. Biello, Vice-President and Editor-in-Chief of Health-Related Professions. As this is my first publication, I was more than a little apprehensive at the onset. However, her support and timely advice helped me to complete this book with limited stress, and, to my surprise, I enjoyed myself immensely every step of the way.

I would also like to thank my instructors, who provided me with a comprehensive and thought-provoking education in radiography and science. I owe a special thanks to Mr. Steven Ahrenstein, instructor of Computed Tomography at the C.W. Post Campus of Long Island University.

The appearance of the high-quality CT images in this book is made possible through the generosity of Dr. Donald Fagelman and Great Neck Imaging, P.C., in Great Neck, New York. Sincere appreciation is extended to Dr. Fagelman and the staff of Great Neck Imaging for their assistance and support.

I also extend a word of thanks to my colleagues at the C.W. Post Campus of Long Island University for their encouragement throughout the development and publication of this book. To the director of the Radiologic Technology Program, Mr. James F. Joyce, I do not think that it is possible to completely thank you for all that you have done for me. In the 8 years that we have known each other, you have been my teacher, mentor, colleague, and most importantly, a true friend. I thank you.

To my students, I can say only that words cannot express the gratitude that I owe to all of you. Your curiosity, insight, and enthusiasm make it all worthwhile. I will do my best to continue to earn the distinct honor of having you call me "teacher."

I've dedicated this book to my parents, as they both struggled and sacrificed a great deal to help provide me with an education. Mom and Dad, all you ever asked for in return was for me to be happy and successful in my endeavors. Rather than thank you again, let me instead promise to constantly strive for excellence in the career that your love and support made possible for me.

Finally, I am forever indebted to Ms. Christine O'Rourke. As with all aspects of our life together, this book is a joint accomplishment. It would not have been possible without you. You are the best friend I could ever hope for, and your love shows me that all things are possible. Thank you.

Contents

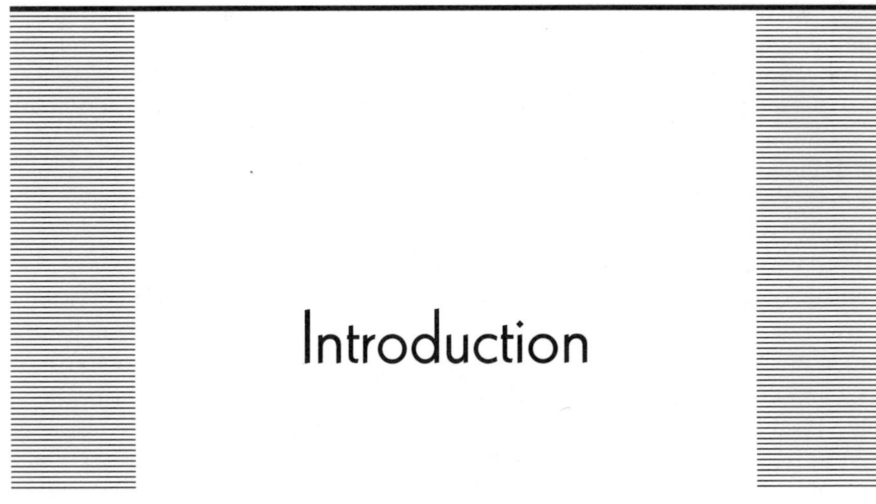

Introduction

The ARRT Advanced-Level Examination in Computed Tomography

The American Registry of Radiologic Technologists (ARRT) advanced-level examination in computed tomography (CT) was first offered in March of 1995. It was designed to provide the technologist with an opportunity to become registered specifically in CT. The CT registry is a 150-question, multiple-choice examination covering three major subject areas in the following manner:

Topic	Number of Questions
Patient Care	30
Imaging Procedures	75
Physics and Instrumentation	45

Complete content specifications, which provide a more extensive look at the subject matter, are available through the ARRT. The ARRT offers the examination on the third Thursday of March, July, and October. The ARRT has strict deadlines for examination application, and interested persons should contact the ARRT as soon as possible.

Using This Review Book

Registry Review in Computed Tomography was developed shortly after I successfully completed the CT registry examination in March of 1995. Questions generated herein resemble those that appeared on that first examination.

This book is designed for two different groups of examination applicants, those with clinical experience and those without. For the established CT technologist, the review questions help bridge the gap between clinical experience and cognitive knowledge. Those who are experienced in CT are already familiar with much of the subject matter covered. This review book allows such persons to answer questions concerning the principles and procedures that are put into practice each day. Because the CT registry is an "advanced-level" examination, some of the subject matter may exceed the standard responsibilities of the staff CT technologist. Practical experience in CT does not eliminate the need for study and preparation to achieve success on this examination. Use of this book in conjunction with some additional reference materials should adequately prepare the student for the CT registry examination.

Many examinees may be using the advanced-level examination in CT as a vehicle toward developing a career in CT. This second group of test applicants may have little or no experience in CT. Such students have a significantly larger amount of work ahead and should review several of the textbooks listed as references in the Appendix during the initial stages of preparation. It is important to review the physical principles of CT imaging along with the many clinical applications such as patient care, scanning protocols, cross-sectional anatomy, and the identification of pathologic conditions on the CT image. This book then serves as an invaluable tool in testing newly acquired knowledge and in practicing "registry-type" questions.

The best way to reap benefits from review books such as this one is to concentrate on the questions that are answered incorrectly. It is not sufficient to simply grade each examination and calculate a score to determine whether a student passed the examination. Each correct answer should be looked up, the brief explanation should be read, and the topic should be further reviewed in the reference cited.

Text Format

Chapters 1 through 4 are four full-length practice examinations. Each examination contains 150 multiple-choice questions. The topics for questions follow the content specifications of the ARRT advanced-level examination in CT. Each practice examination is weighted concerning subject area in a similar manner to that of the ARRT examination.

Chapters 5 through 8 contain the correct answers to each examination. A brief explanation accompanies each correct answer, followed by a reference, which contains detailed information on the topic.

Many of the questions in each examination pertain to a particular CT image. All the information provided by the image should be used when attempting to correctly answer these questions.

Study Habits/Test-Taking Techniques

Each student preparing to take the ARRT advanced-level examination in CT is a registered or licensed radiologic technologist who has already successfully completed a registry examination in the radiologic sciences. Such students have experience with taking standardized examinations; however, the following study tips should be useful reminders:

1. Do not wait until the last minute to prepare. Start with a general text in the physical principles of CT and progress through the multitude of clinical applications of CT. Because a large percentage of the examination pertains to cross-sectional anatomy, do not rely only on practical experience in this area. Carefully review a text containing CT images with detailed cross-sectional anatomy that is well-labeled. This book should not be used as the sole preparatory tool for the ARRT examination. It is not a "quick-fix" and does not make up for lack of adequate research and study.

2. Practice time management skills. This is equally important during preparation and during the examination. Three hours are allotted to complete 150 questions. This should be more than sufficient. Bring a watch to the testing center and follow the standard rule of not spending too much time on any one question.

3. Zero in on the correct answer. Success on standardized examinations lies in the ability not only to choose the correct answer but also to identify the incorrect ones. The process of elimination is a valued asset when answering a multiple-choice question. Carefully examine each answer and eliminate those that are obviously incorrect. This often narrows the possible choices and improves the chances when guessing becomes a necessity.

4. Have confidence. You are in the midst of a successful career in medical imaging. Your interest in the field and your dedication to continued learning have brought you here to this advanced-level examination. Have confidence in your ability and put some faith in your preparation and experience—you know the material; relax and simply tap into this knowledge.

CHAPTER 1

Simulated Exam One

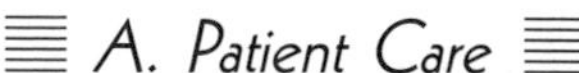

A. Patient Care

1. The normal range of respiration for an adult is
   a. 5–10 breaths per minute
   b. 12–20 breaths per minute
   c. 20–30 breaths per minute
   d. 35–50 breaths per minute

2. Which of the following is a parenteral route of medication administration?
   a. sublingual
   b. intramuscular
   c. transdermal
   d. oral

3. The preparation for a contrast-enhanced CT exam of a patient with prior allergic reaction to iodinated contrast media may include
   a. premedication with steroids and antihistamines
   b. administration of a negative contrast agent
   c. increase in fluids for 24 hours before the examination
   d. refraining from urination for 2 hours before the examination

4. A patient in shock may exhibit which of the following symptoms:
   a. tachycardia
   b. rapid, shallow breathing
   c. cyanosis
   d. all of the above

5. Which of the following infection control techniques is required at the site of an intravenous injection of iodinated contrast media?
   a. contact isolation
   b. surgical asepsis
   c. medical asepsis
   d. enteric precautions

6. A common site for the intravenous injection of iodinated contrast media is the

a. cephalic vein
b. antecubital vein
c. basilic vein
d. all of the above

7. Which of the following technical factors exhibits a direct effect on patient dose?

a. matrix size
b. algorithm
c. milliampere-seconds (mAs)
d. window level

8. Prior to an intravenous injection of iodinated contrast material, the patient should be questioned regarding

1. renal function
2. allergic history
3. cardiac history

a. 1 only
b. 2 only
c. 3 only
d. 1, 2, and 3

9. Used in determining the biologic effect of iodinated contrast media, the term _______________ refers to the number of ions formed when a substance dissociates in solution.

a. solubility
b. osmolality
c. concentration
d. iodination

10. Which of the following laboratory values can be used to evaluate the renal function of a patient?

a. blood urea nitrogen (BUN)
b. partial thromboplastin time
c. creatinine
d. both a and c

11. A(n) _______________ infection is one that patients acquire during their stay in a health care institution.

a. blood-borne
b. nosocomial
c. iatrogenic
d. staphylococcal

12. During CT examinations, patients should be shielded above and below because of

a. the rotational nature of the x-ray tube
b. extremely high kilovolt peak (kVp) techniques
c. lack of filtration of the CT beam
d. reduced collimation of the CT beam

13. Which of the following would be best suited for intravenous injection of contrast material with a power injector?

a. a butterfly needle
b. a central venous line
c. a 23-gauge spinal needle
d. an angiocatheter

14. A(n) _______________ contrast material may be described as one that does not dissociate into charged particles in solution.

a. neutral
b. non-ionic
c. osmolar
d. ionic

15. Thorough explanation of the CT procedure and proper communication with the patient is vital in ensuring that

1. breathing instructions are properly followed
2. misregistration does not occur
3. patient anxiety is kept at a minimum

a. 1 and 2 only
b. 1 and 3 only
c. 2 and 3 only
d. 1, 2, and 3

16. The lumen of needles used for the injection of contrast media varies in diameter. The unit used to describe this diameter is called

a. length
b. cubic centimeter (cc)
c. gauge
d. pounds per square inch (psi)

17. Direct contraindications to iodinated contrast material administration include

1. prior life-threatening reaction to iodinated contrast material
2. multiple myeloma
3. allergies to penicillin

a. 1 only
b. 1 and 2 only
c. 1 and 3 only
d. 1, 2, and 3

18. Which of the following is an accurate method of verifying patient identity?

a. calling patients by their full names
b. checking the name listed on the medical record
c. examining the patient's wrist identification band
d. all of the above

19. Advantages of automatic power injectors over the manual bolus method of intravenous contrast administration include

1. increased tissue enhancement due to faster injection times
2. uniform contrast administration over the entire length of the study
3. decreased volume of contrast administered

a. 1 only
b. 3 only
c. 1 and 2 only
d. 2 and 3 only

20. The average range for normal adult blood urea nitrogen (BUN) levels is approximately

a. 1–4 mg/dL
b. 5–20 mg/dL
c. 23–30 mg/dL
d. 45–60mg/dL

21. Which of the following terms describes a condition in which cerebral ischemia is caused by systemic hypotension?

a. vasovagal reaction
b. myocardial infarction
c. transient ischemic attack
d. hydrocephalus

22. Which of the following interactions between x-ray beam and matter results in the largest amount of patient dose?

a. characteristic
b. Compton scatter
c. bremsstrahlung
d. photoelectric effect

23. Examples of mild adverse reactions to iodinated intravenous contrast media may include

1. nausea
2. dyspnea
3. warm, flushed sensation

a. 1 only
b. 1 and 2 only
c. 1 and 3 only
d. 2 and 3 only

24. During which of the following CT procedures is the patient required to give informed consent?

a. noncontrast chest examination
b. radiation planning study of the prostate
c. three-dimensional reconstruction of the hip
d. abdomen scan with intravenous contrast

25. ________________ is a medication commonly administered to sedate small children undergoing CT examinations.

a. Chloral hydrate
b. Lithium
c. Diazepam (Valium)
d. Secobarbital sodium (Seconal Sodium)

26. Which of the following are included as basic types of iodinated contrast media?

1. iothalamate
2. diatrizoate
3. metrizoate

a. 2 only
b. 3 only
c. 1 and 3 only
d. 1, 2, and 3

27. Which of the following is not a category of isolation technique?

a. enteric precautions
b. gram-negative isolation
c. contact isolation
d. strict isolation

28. Which of the following correctly states the difference between ionic and non-ionic iodinated contrast material?

a. Non-ionic contrast media have a higher osmolality than ionic media.
b. Ionic contrast media contain iodine, whereas non-ionic contrast media do not.
c. Non-ionic contrast media have a lower osmolality than ionic media.
d. Ionic contrast media involve a lower incidence of adverse reactions than non-ionic contrast media.

29. Which of the following terms is used to describe the intravenous injection of medication or contrast agent in one complete dose over a short period of time?

a. infusion
b. bolus
c. intravenous drip
d. Infuse-A-Port

30. An intrathecal injection before a CT examination of the lumbar spine places iodinated contrast material directly into the

a. subarachnoid space
b. dura mater
c. vertebral foramen
d. subdural space

B. Imaging Procedures

31. Accurate demonstration of ________________ would most likely require the intravenous injection of an iodinated contrast medium during a CT study of the chest.

a. bronchiectasis
b. pneumonia
c. mediastinal lymphadenopathy
d. a pulmonary nodule

32. Abnormalities of the middle and inner ear may be best demonstrated using CT sections of

a. 1–2 mm
b. 3–4 mm
c. 5 mm
d. 10 mm

33. Which of the following is not a portion of the small bowel?

a. duodenum
b. jejunum
c. ileum
d. cecum

34. Axial CT sections of the lumbar spine for intervertebral disk evaluation should be acquired with the plane of imaging

a. perpendicular to the transverse plane of the patient
b. parallel to the plane of the intervertebral disk spaces
c. parallel to the transverse plane of the patient
d. perpendicular to the coronal plane of the patient

Questions 35–36 refer to Figure 1–1.

35. Number 5 corresponds to which of the following?

a. gallbladder
b. inferior vena cava
c. descending aorta
d. right adrenal gland

36. Number 3 corresponds to which of the following?

a. spleen
b. small bowel
c. descending colon
d. left kidney

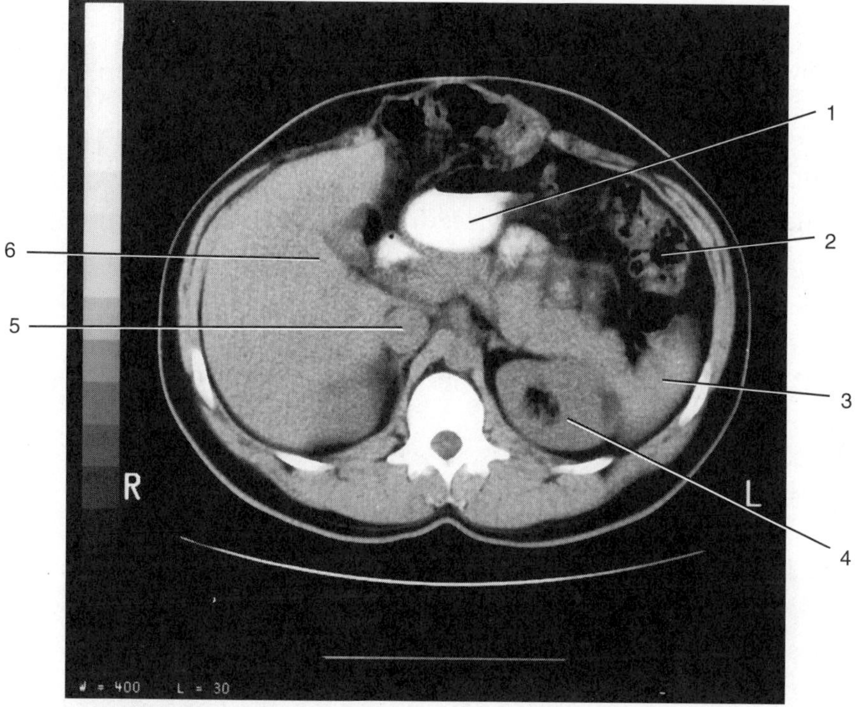

Figure 1–1.

37. Which of the following is a typical protocol for a CT study of the brain for a patient with a history of dizziness?

a. 10- × 10-mm sections from the skull base to the vertex

b. 10- × 10-mm sections from the skull base to the posterior fossa

c. 5- × 5-mm sections through the posterior fossa, 10 mm × 10 mm to the vertex

d. 1.5- × 1.5-mm sections from the skull base to the vertex

38. A ______________ is a benign, highly vascular mass commonly found in the liver.

a. hematoid

b. vasculoma

c. hemogenic carcinoma

d. hemangioma

39. Simple cysts of the kidney have average attenuation values in the range of

a. −40 to 0 Hounsfield units

b. 0 to +20 Hounsfield units

c. +30 to +50 Hounsfield units

d. more than +60 Hounsfield units

Questions 40–42 refer to Figure 1–2.

40. Number 2 corresponds to which of the following?

a. left ovary
b. bladder
c. sigmoid colon
d. uterus

41. Number 4 corresponds to which of the following?

a. left ovary
b. bladder
c. sigmoid colon
d. uterus

42. Number 5 corresponds to which of the following?

a. left ovary
b. bladder
c. sigmoid colon
d. uterus

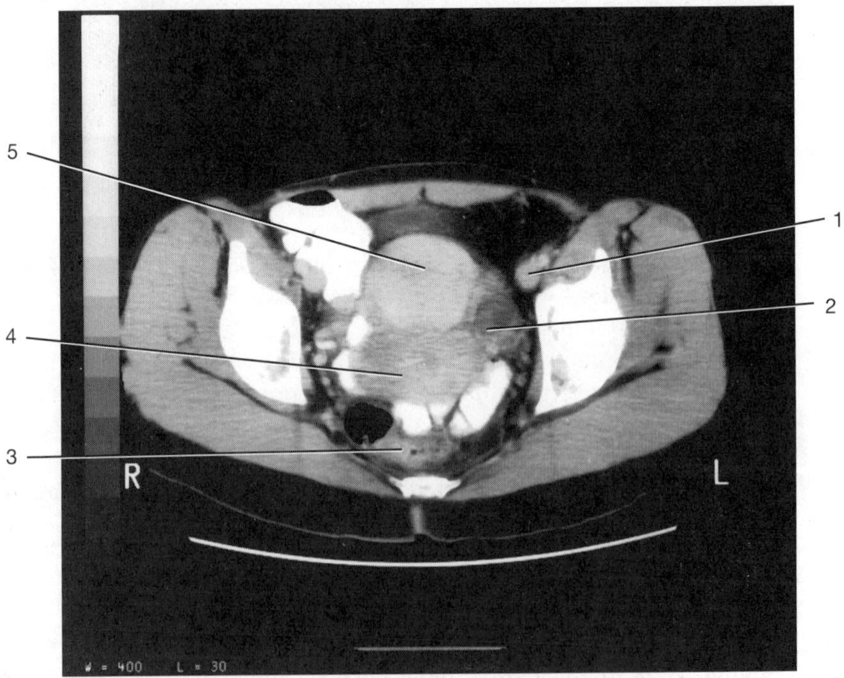

Figure 1–2.

43. The proper scan field of view (SFOV) for a CT of the abdomen of a patient who measures 42 cm is

a. head (25 cm)
b. small (25 cm)
c. medium (35 cm)
d. large (48 cm)

44. CT images of the chest should be acquired with the patient

a. at full inspiration
b. breathing quietly
c. at full expiration
d. breathing normally

45. Which of the following protocols would provide the best image quality for a three-dimensional disarticulation study of the hip?

a. 10- × 15-mm sections, standard algorithm
b. 10- × 10-mm sections, bone algorithm
c. 1.5- × 1.0-mm sections, bone algorithm
d. 5- × 7-mm sections, standard algorithm

46. Which of the following patient positions is best suited for CT evaluation of the chest?

a. prone
b. left lateral decubitus
c. right lateral decubitus
d. supine

47. During a spiral or helical CT examination, the scanner acquires data

a. continuously as the patient travels through the gantry
b. one section at a time
c. in the form of a complete volumetric data set
d. both a and c

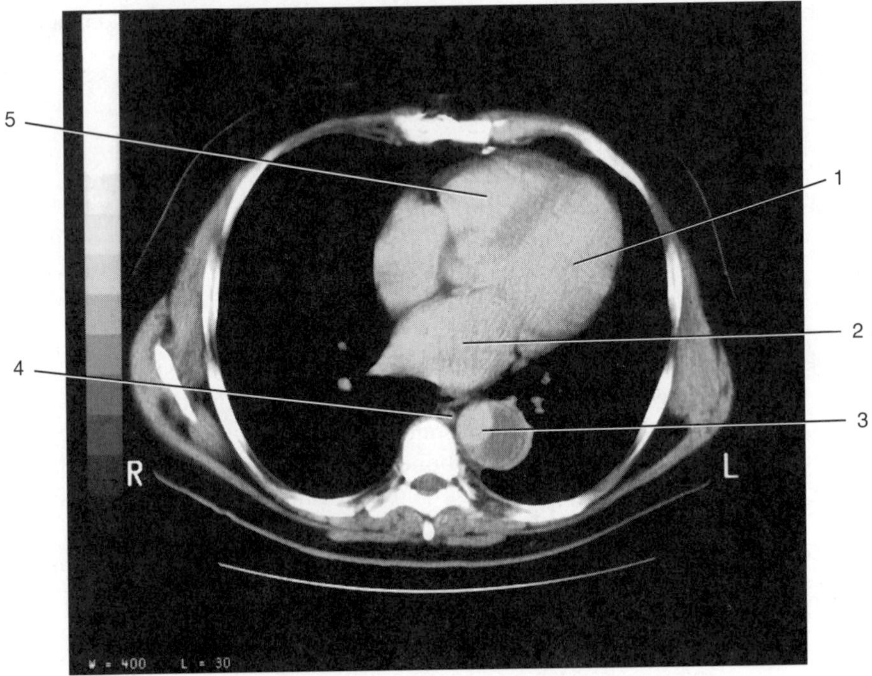

Figure 1–3.

Questions 48–50 refer to Figure 1–3.

48. Number 5 corresponds to which of the following?

a. left atrium
b. right ventricle
c. ascending aorta
d. descending aorta

49. Which number corresponds to the left atrium?

a. 1
b. 2
c. 3
d. 4

50. Number 4 corresponds to which of the following?

a. azygos vein
b. superior vena cava
c. left ventricle
d. right atrium

51. A complete CT study of the orbits should include

a. 10- × 10-mm axial sections only
b. 10- × 10-mm axial and coronal sections
c. 3- × 3-mm coronal sections only
d. 3- × 3-mm axial and coronal sections

52. Dynamic CT studies involve rapid bolus contrast administration followed by immediate data acquisition with which of the following parameter characteristics?

a. long interscan delays
b. noncontiguous sections with wide interspaces
c. rapidly scanned sections with short interscan delays
d. detail algorithm

53. Which of the following contrast media may be used during the CT evaluation of the gastrointestinal tract?

1. diatrizoate meglumine (Gastrografin)
2. effervescent agents
3. iopamidol (Isovue)

a. 1 only
b. 1 and 3 only
c. 2 and 3 only
d. 1, 2, and 3

Questions 54–56 refer to Figure 1–4.

54. Which number corresponds to the anterior horn of the lateral ventricle?

a. 1
b. 5
c. 3
d. 2

55. Number 3 corresponds to which of the following?

a. caudate nucleus
b. thalamus
c. third ventricle
d. pineal gland

56. Which number corresponds to the septum pellucidum?

a. 2
b. 3
c. 4
d. 5

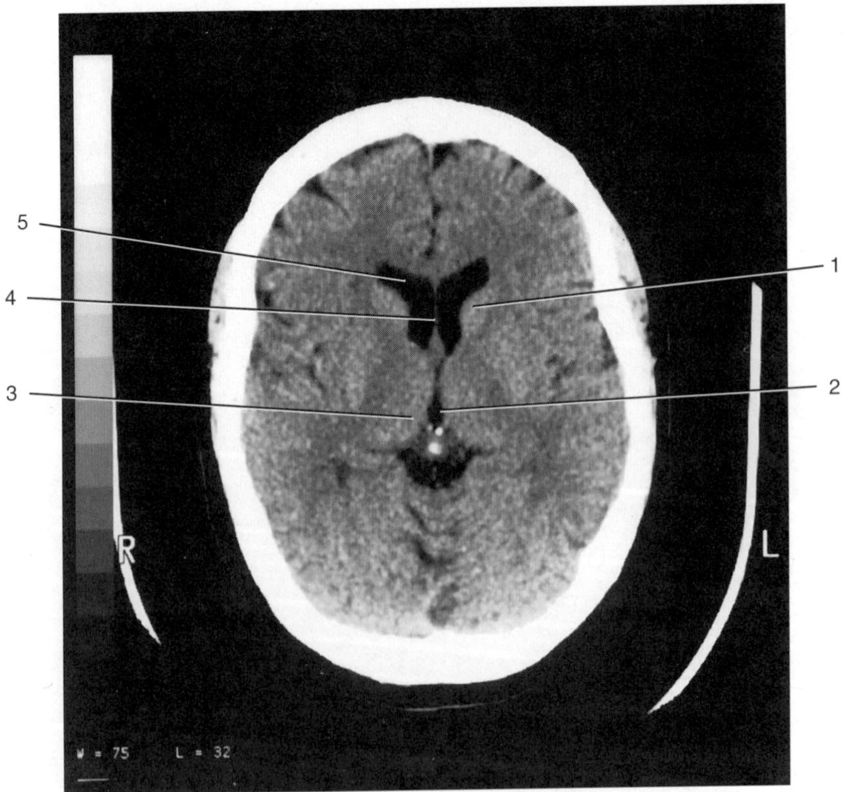

Figure 1–4.

57. Complete CT examinations of the chest for investigation of bronchogenic carcinoma should include sections from the

a. mandible through the liver
b. apices to the diaphragm
c. top of the apices through the liver
d. clavicles through the adrenals

58. Which of the following contrast administration techniques should be used for a general CT survey of the abdomen?

1. 400–600 mL of oral contrast administered 45–90 minutes before the examination
2. 300 mL of oral contrast administered immediately before the examination
3. a 700-mL–900-mL enema given immediately before the examination

a. 1 only
b. 1 and 2 only
c. 1 and 3 only
d. 1, 2, and 3

59. The scout (localizer) performed for a CT of the brain should be which of the following projections?

a. anteroposterior
b. submentovertex
c. lateral
d. posteroanterior

Questions 60–63 refer to Figure 1–5.

60. Number 6 corresponds to which of the following pathologic processes?

a. renal stone
b. hepatic abscess
c. appendicolith
d. cholelithiasis

61. Which number corresponds to the superior mesenteric vein?

a. 3
b. 5
c. 1
d. 2

62. Number 4 corresponds to which of the following?

a. duodenum
b. pancreas
c. jejunum
d. gallbladder

63. Which of the following window width and level settings were used to display the image?

a. L = –700, W = 2000
b. L = +250, W = 800
c. L = +50, W = 400
d. L = +70, W = 150

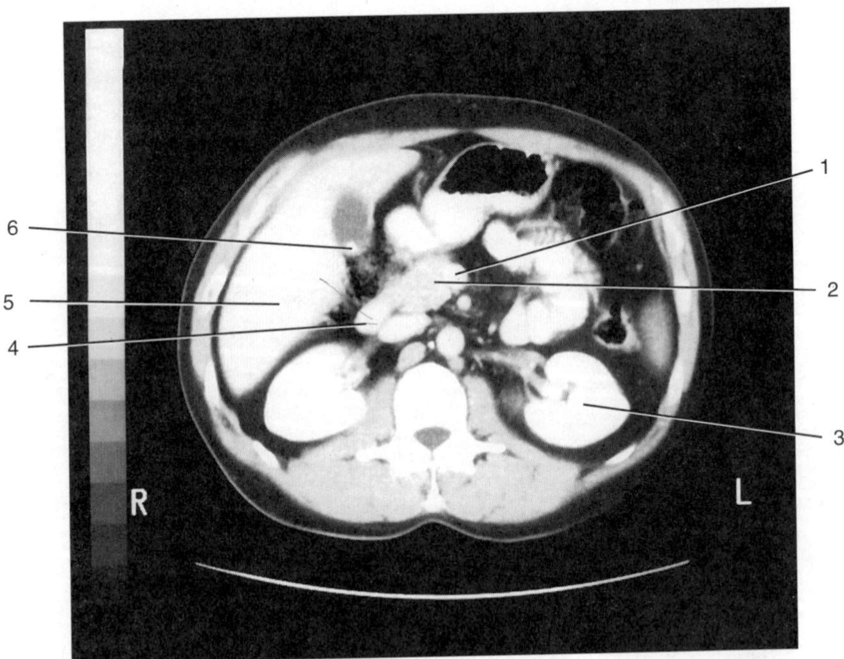

Figure 1–5.

64. The portion of the nephron that filters unwanted materials from the blood plasma is called the

a. afferent arteriole
b. proximal tubule
c. efferent arteriole
d. glomerulus

65. The adult spinal cord ends at what vertebral level?

a. T11–T12
b. L1–L2
c. L3–L4
d. superior portion of the coccyx

66. During a complete CT scan of the pelvis, sections should be obtained from the

a. iliac crests to the pubic symphysis
b. kidneys through the bladder
c. bottom of the kidneys to the pubic symphysis
d. iliac crests to the lesser trochanter

67. The purpose of intravenous contrast administration during a CT study is to

1. increase the contrast of adjacent structures
2. increase examination cost to the patient
3. increase beam attenuation of enhanced structures

a. 1 only
b. 1 and 3 only
c. 2 and 3 only
d. 3 only

68. The pituitary gland is best demonstrated during CT with which of the following imaging planes?

a. axial
b. coronal
c. sagittal
d. transaxial

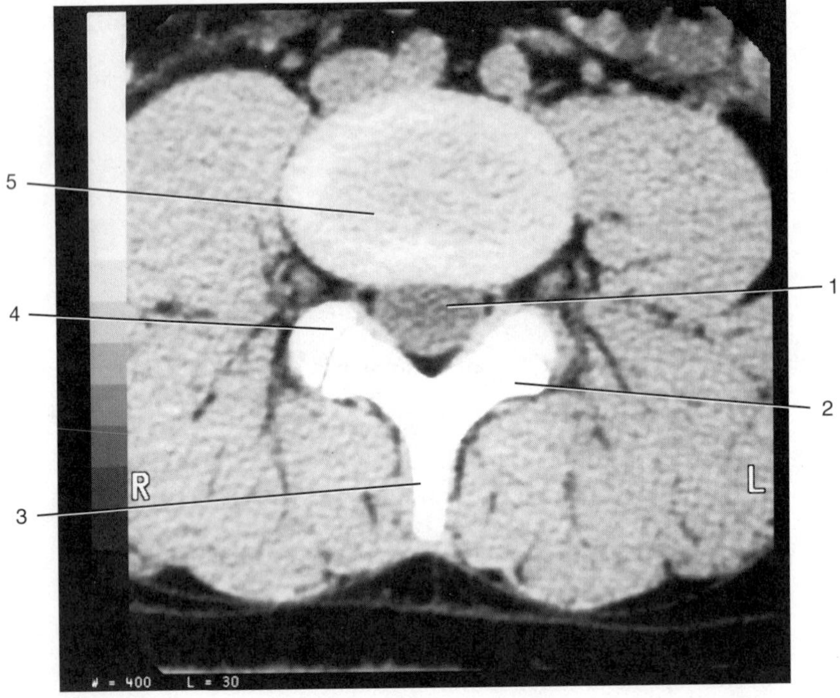

Figure 1–6.

Questions 69–71 refer to Figure 1–6.

69. Which number corresponds to the lamina?

a. 1
b. 2
c. 3
d. 4

70. Number 1 corresponds to which of the following?

a. inferior vena cava
b. ligamentum flavum
c. cauda equina
d. nucleus pulposus

71. Which of the following technical scan factors were used to form this image?

1. plane of imaging parallel to disk space
2. narrow section thickness
3. bone algorithm

a. 1 only
b. 1 and 2 only
c. 2 and 3 only
d. 1, 2, and 3

72. The portion of the male reproductive system that stores most of the mature spermatozoa is the

a. seminal vesicles
b. vas deferens
c. testes
d. prostate gland

73. During CT examination of the larynx, the patient is often instructed to phonate the letter E in order to properly evaluate the

a. epiglottis
b. uvula
c. trachea
d. vocal cords

74. The muscular contraction that propels material through the digestive tract is called

a. mastication
b. phagocytosis
c. peristalsis
d. deglutition

75. Which of the following paranasal sinuses is usually the last to fully develop?

a. frontal
b. ethmoidal
c. sphenoidal
d. maxillary

76. Which of the following scan parameters is commonly used during a radiation planning CT study of the prostate gland?

1. The patient is placed on a flat tabletop.
2. A small display field of view (DFOV) is used to include only the prostate gland.
3. The CT scan is performed with the patient in the exact position to be used for radiation treatment.

a. 1 only
b. 1 and 3 only
c. 2 and 3 only
d. 1, 2, and 3

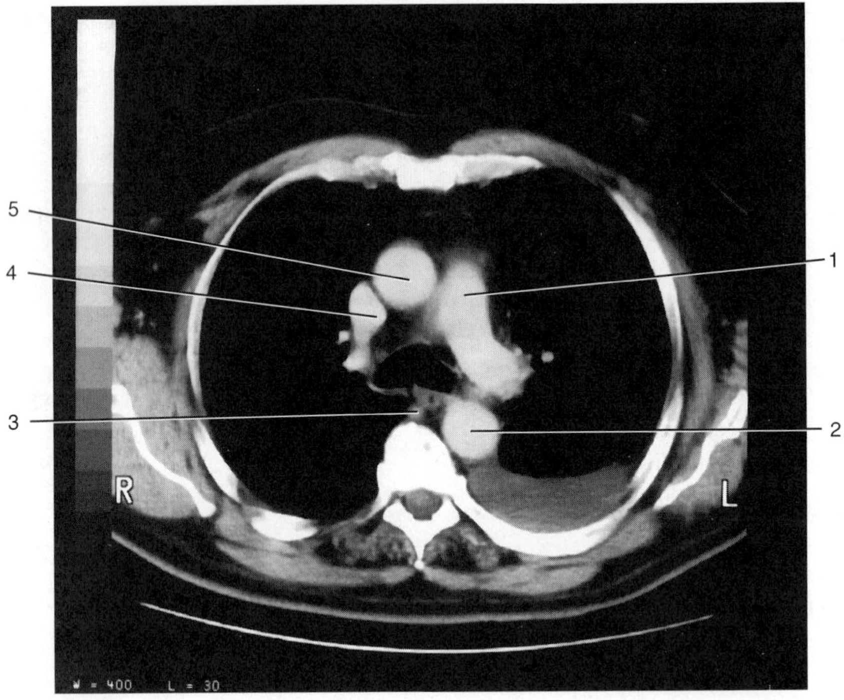

Figure 1–7.

Questions 77–79 refer to Figure 1–7.

77. Number 1 corresponds to which of the following?

a. left pulmonary artery
b. ascending aorta
c. inferior vena cava
d. descending aorta

78. Which number corresponds to the superior vena cava?

a. 4
b. 1
c. 2
d. 3

79. The abnormal density located in the posterior portion of the left lung field has an average attenuation value of +5.0 Hounsfield units. This density most likely represents

a. pneumothorax
b. hemothorax
c. atelectasis
d. pleural effusion

80. The third ventricle of the brain communicates with the fourth ventricle through the

a. anterior commissure
b. septum pellucidum
c. cerebral aqueduct
d. fornix

81. Differentiation between the duodenum and head of the pancreas is best accomplished with

1. oral contrast administered 30–45 minutes before scanning
2. precontrast and postcontrast images of the abdomen
3. the patient placed in the right lateral decubitus position before scanning

a. 1 only
b. 1 and 3 only
c. 2 and 3 only
d. 1, 2, and 3

82. A glioma is a general term used to describe a group of primary tumors. Consisting of malignant glial cells, gliomas occur in the

a. oral cavity
b. kidney
c. brain
d. liver

83. The excretion half-time of intravenous iodinated contrast media in a patient with normal renal function is between

a. 1 and 2 hours
b. 18 and 24 hours
c. 1 and 2 days
d. 5 and 7 days

84. The plane that passes vertically through the midline of the body, dividing it into equal anterior and posterior portions, is referred to as

a. orthogonal
b. axial
c. midsagittal
d. midcoronal

85. ______________ refers to an excessive amount of nitrogenous materials in the blood and is a symptom of renal failure.

a. Hydronephrosis
b. Azotemia
c. Oliguria
d. Diuresis

86. A common formula used to calculate the dosage of intravenous iodinated contrast material in the pediatric patient is

a. 3 mg/kg body weight
b. 5 mL/lb body weight
c. 1 mL/lb body weight
d. 100 mL in patients weighing over 10 lb

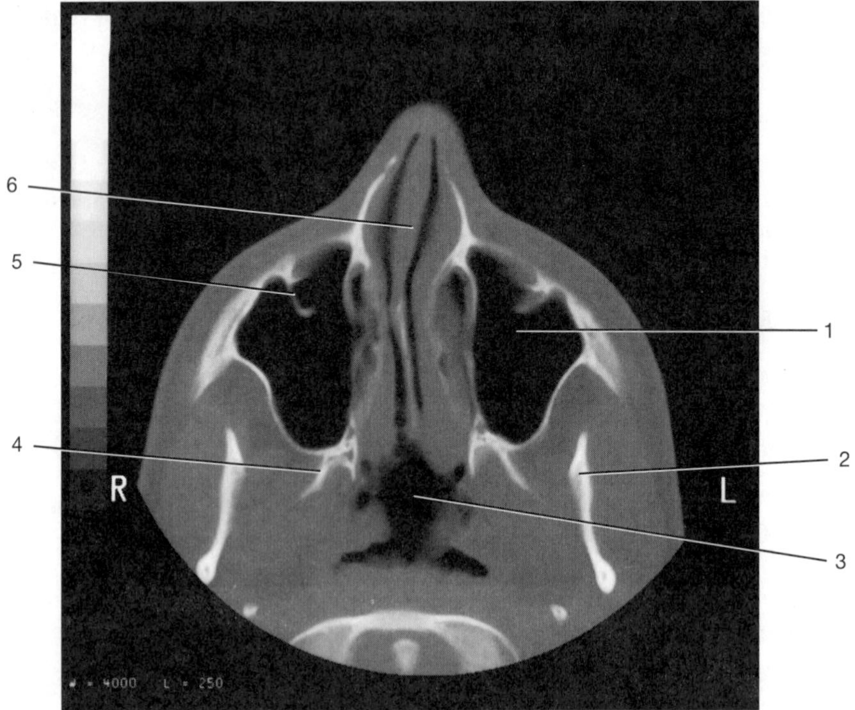

Figure 1–8.

Questions 87–90 refer to Figure 1–8.

87. During a complete CT study, the paranasal sinuses shown in the image should also be scanned in which of the following planes?
   a. axial
   b. sagittal
   c. orthogonal
   d. coronal

88. Number 3 corresponds to which of the following?
   a. nasopharynx
   b. sphenoid sinus
   c. ethmoid sinus
   d. trachea

89. Which of the following numbers corresponds to the right lateral pterygoid plate?
   a. 4
   b. 2
   c. 3
   d. 5

90. Which of the following clinical findings best describes the abnormal anatomic condition labeled as number 6?

a. mucosal thickening
b. deviated septum
c. sinusitis
d. retropharyngeal hematoma

91. Which of the following sets of section width and incrementation is best suited for a CT examination of the cervical spine to rule out intervertebral disk herniation?

a. 5 × 5 mm
b. 3 × 3 mm
c. 5 × 7 mm
d. 10 × 10 mm

92. During which of the following phases of intravenous contrast administration should CT images of the liver be acquired?

1. bolus phase
2. nonequilibrium phase
3. equilibrium phase

a. 1 only
b. 2 only
c. 1 and 2 only
d. 1, 2, and 3

93. The mediastinum includes which of the following anatomic structures?

1. superior vena cava
2. stomach
3. ascending aorta

a. 1 only
b. 1 and 2 only
c. 1 and 3 only
d. 1, 2, and 3

Questions 94–97 refer to Figure 1–9.

94. Which of the following patient positions may have been used to produce this scout image of the head?
   a. supine
   b. lateral
   c. prone
   d. both a and c

95. Number 1 corresponds to which of the following?
   a. lateral pterygoid plate
   b. styloid process
   c. rostrum
   d. posterior clinoid process

96. Number 3 corresponds to which of the following?
   a. external auditory meatus
   b. foramen rotundum
   c. foramen ovale
   d. mastoid air cells

97. The scout image shown could be used as a localizer to plan portions of CT examinations for which of the following?
   1. paranasal sinuses
   2. pituitary
   3. internal auditory canals
      a. 1 only
      b. 1 and 2 only
      c. 2 and 3 only
      d. 1, 2, and 3

98. Which of the following is not a necessary technique when performing a CT examination of an extremity to rule out a fracture?
   a. inclusion of a normal extremity when possible for comparison
   b. performance of a contiguous study consisting of narrow section width
   c. administration of intravenous contrast
   d. recording of images at bone window settings

99. During a CT examination of the abdomen, intravenous contrast is indicated and is administered with the aid of an automatic injector. Which of the following ranges of flow rates should be used?
   a. 0.2–1.0 mL/sec
   b. 1.0–3.0 mL/sec
   c. 4.0–6.0 mL/sec
   d. 7.0–10.0 mL/sec

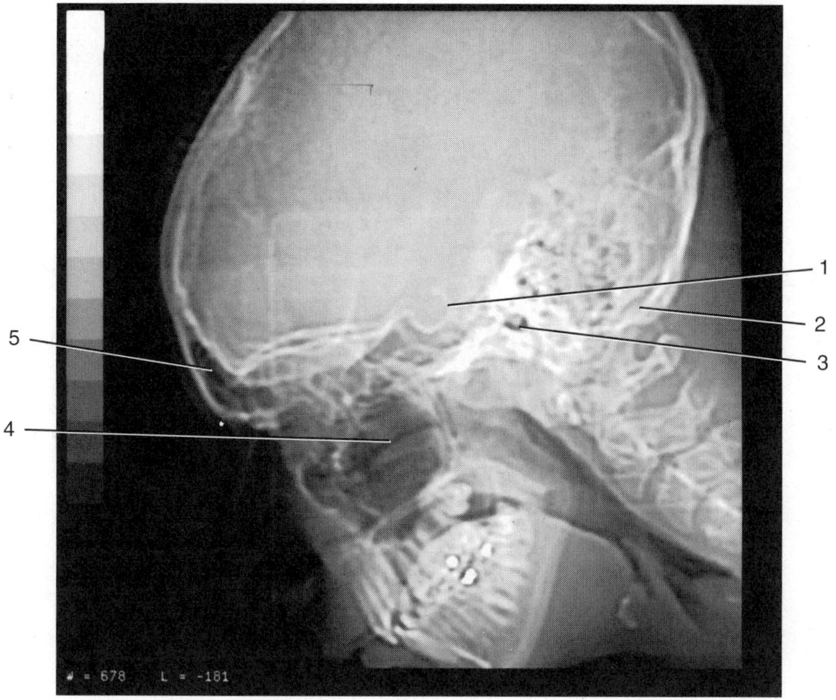

Figure 1–9.

100. Percutaneous drainage under CT guidance may be used for the aspiration of which of the following pathologic processes?

a. chronic subdural hematoma
b. hydrocephalus
c. abdominal abscess
d. dissecting aortic aneurysm

101. An enema is indicated before a CT examination of the pelvis to administer positive contrast material into the large bowel. Which of the following doses is sufficient to opacify the rectosigmoid region?

a. 150–250 mL
b. 300–500 mL → to fill lg bowel.
c. 500–750 mL
d. 900–1100 mL

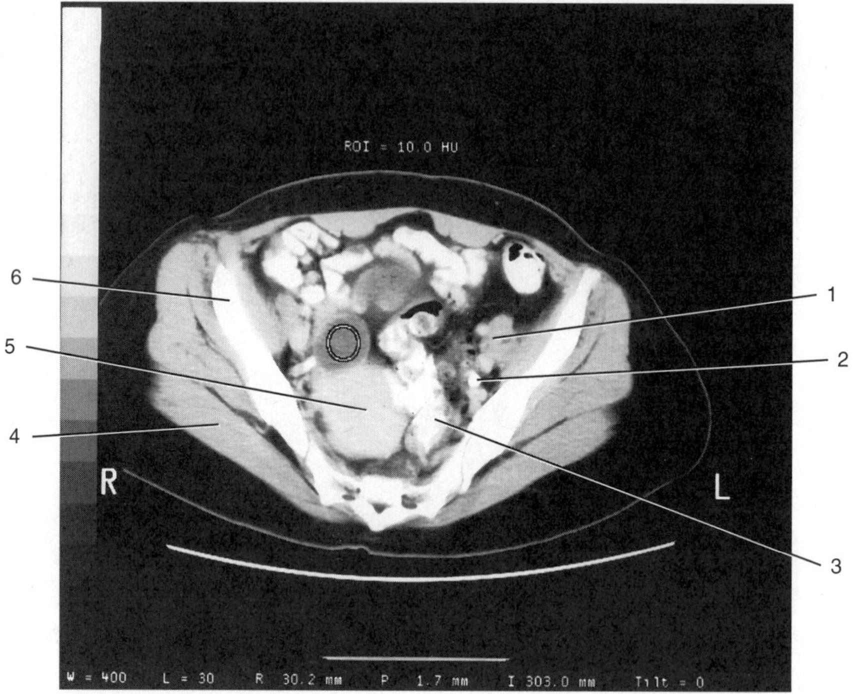

Figure 1–10.

Questions 102–105 refer to Figure 1–10.

102. The region of interest measurement in the figure has an average Hounsfield value of +10. When its position in this female pelvis is considered, this density most likely represents a

a. fibroid uterus
b. ovarian cyst
c. diverticular abscess
d. endometrial tumor

103. Number 5 corresponds to which of the following?

a. right ovary
b. bladder
c. uterus
d. prostate gland

104. Number 1 corresponds to which of the following?

a. iliacus muscle
b. gluteus minimus muscle
c. superior gluteal artery
d. psoas major muscle

105. Which number corresponds to the ilium?

a. 3
b. 6
c. 4
d. 2

C. Physics and Instrumentation

106. Partial volume averaging on the CT image may be decreased by

a. increasing matrix size
b. decreasing matrix size
c. increasing slice thickness
d. decreasing slice thickness

107. The loss of anatomic information between contiguous sections due to inconsistent patient breathing is called

a. cupping artifact
b. misregistration
c. overshoot artifact
d. out-of-field artifact

108. A CT image is formed in part by projecting back all of the attenuation values recorded during data acquisition onto a

a. pixel
b. voxel
c. matrix
d. reformat

109. What is the dimension of each pixel in an image with a 512- × 512-mm matrix and a DFOV equaling 25.6 cm?

a. 0.5 mm
b. 0.5 cm
c. 0.05 cm
d. both a and c

110. The following formula is used to calculate the linear attenuation coefficient: $I = I_0e^{-\mu x}$ where x equals

a. Euler's constant
b. absorber thickness
c. the unknown
d. transmitted photons

111. First-generation CT scanners used a method of data acquisition based on a _____________ principle.

a. multiplanar
b. rotation only
c. translate–rotate
d. transaxial

112. CT numbers are usually provided in the form of

a. Hounsfield units
b. electromagnetic interference numbers
c. Cormacks
d. μ

113. Which of the following may be used for the archival storage of CT images?

1. magnetic tape
2. VHS tape
3. magnetic optical disk

a. 1 only
b. 1 and 3 only
c. 2 and 3 only
d. 1, 2, and 3

114. The reduction in intensity of an x-ray beam as it interacts with matter is termed

a. scatter
b. attenuation
c. transmission
d. luminescence

115. The major disadvantage of the fan-shaped x-ray beams used in modern CT units when compared with "pencil-thin" beams is

a. increased transmission measurements
b. increased patient dose
c. decreased transmission measurements
d. excess tube wear

116. Which of the following is the most common type of noise found in the CT image?

a. statistical noise
b. electronic noise
c. artifactual noise
d. filter noise

117. Scintillation crystals are used exclusively as detectors in _____________ CT scanners.

a. electron beam
b. third-generation
c. fourth-generation
d. spiral

118. A first-generation CT scanner consists of an x-ray tube and two detectors that translate across the patient's head while rotating in 1° increments for a total of

a. 45°
b. 90°
c. 180°
d. 360°

119. Which of the following factors does not affect the dimensions of a voxel?

a. slice thickness
b. matrix size
c. kernel
d. DFOV

120. Areas of a CT image that contain abrupt changes in tissue density are electronically represented by which of the following?

a. positive CT numbers
b. high spatial frequencies
c. negative CT numbers
d. low spatial frequencies

121. The CT "window" controls the ______________ of the CT image.

a. density and detail
b. spatial and contrast resolution
c. contrast and brightness
d. attenuation coefficient and Hounsfield value

122. Which of the following is an analytic form of image reconstruction?

1. iterative technique
2. Fourier reconstruction
3. filtered back-projection

a. 1 only
b. 1 and 2 only
c. 2 and 3 only
d. 1, 2, and 3

123. Which of the following archival media is capable of storing the largest number of CT images?

a. floppy disk
b. magnetic tape
c. VHS tape
d. optical disk

124. The term used to describe the relation between the linear attenuation coefficients of an object and the calculated CT numbers is

a. linearity
b. mottle
c. quantum noise
d. spatial resolution

125. The component of the CT scanner responsible for the mathematical calculations of the image reconstruction process is the
   a. Data acquisition system (DAS)
   b. Analog-to-digital converter
   c. Digital-to-analog converter
   d. Array processor

126. Which of the following statements regarding retrospective image reconstruction is false?
   a. The algorithm, matrix size, and DFOV may all be changed.
   b. The slice thickness and SFOV may be changed.
   c. Scan (raw) data must be available.
   d. Retrospective image reconstruction may be used to adjust the center of the displayed image.

127. Which of the following decreases the noise of a CT image?
   a. decrease in dose
   b. decrease in slice thickness
   c. increase in matrix size
   d. decrease in matrix size

128. Increasing the pitch during a spiral CT examination adversely affects the spatial resolution along with which of the following?
   a. axial plane
   b. x axis
   c. y axis
   d. z axis

129. Which of the following statements regarding prepatient collimation is true?
1. An increase in prepatient collimation increases patient dose.
2. Prepatient collimation is used to focus radiation through the section of interest.
3. Prepatient collimation directly controls slice thickness.
   a. 2 only
   b. 3 only
   c. 1 and 2 only
   d. 2 and 3 only

130. When an operator reduces the SFOV for a particular body part, which of the following technical changes occurs?
   a. The displayed image appears larger.
   b. Spatial resolution increases.
   c. A smaller number of detectors are activated.
   d. The displayed image appears smaller.

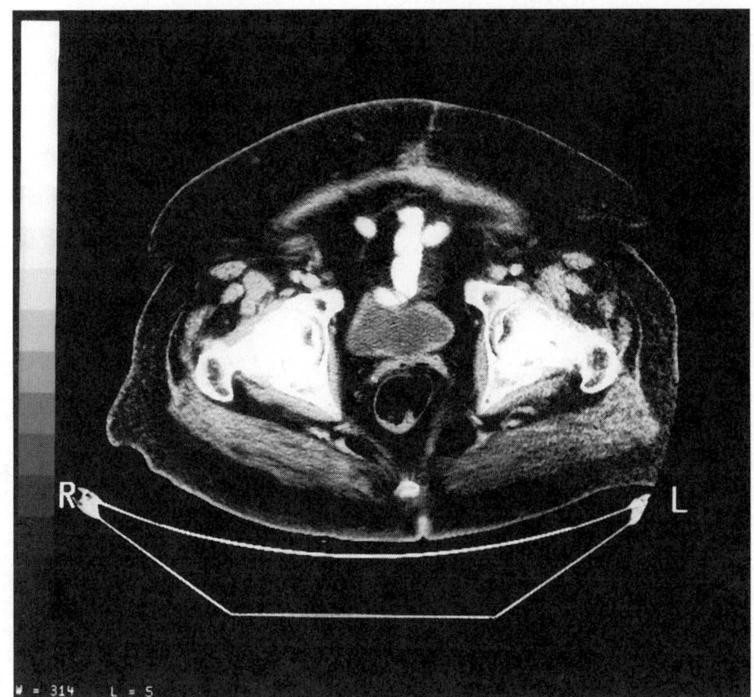

Figure 1–11.

Questions 131–132 refer to Figure 1–11.

131. The grainy appearance of this pelvic image is commonly referred to as

a. tube arcing
b. noise
c. edge gradient
d. partial volume artifact

132. Which of the following is the most likely cause of this inferior image quality?

a. beam hardening
b. detector malfunction
c. insufficient patient dose
d. incorrect SFOV

133. An average CT number value for blood is

a. −20 Hounsfield units
b. +10 Hounsfield units
c. +45 Hounsfield units
d. +100 Hounsfield units

134. Which of the following types of gas is commonly used for gas ionization CT detectors?

a. xenon
b. cadmium tungstate
c. helium
d. nitrogen

Questions 135–136 refer to Figure 1–12.

135. The artifact present on the lateral borders of the image most likely represents which of the following?

a. edge gradient
b. out-of-field artifact
c. tube arcing
d. beam hardening

136. The image was produced using the following parameters: large (full) scan field of view, maximum DFOV (48 cm), 200 mA, 120 kVp, soft-tissue algorithm. Which of the following technical adjustments would reduce the artifact?

a. Switch to a detail or bone algorithm.
b. Use a smaller SFOV.
c. Increase 200 mA to 240 mA and increase 120 kVp to 140 kVp.
d. Center the patient within the SFOV.

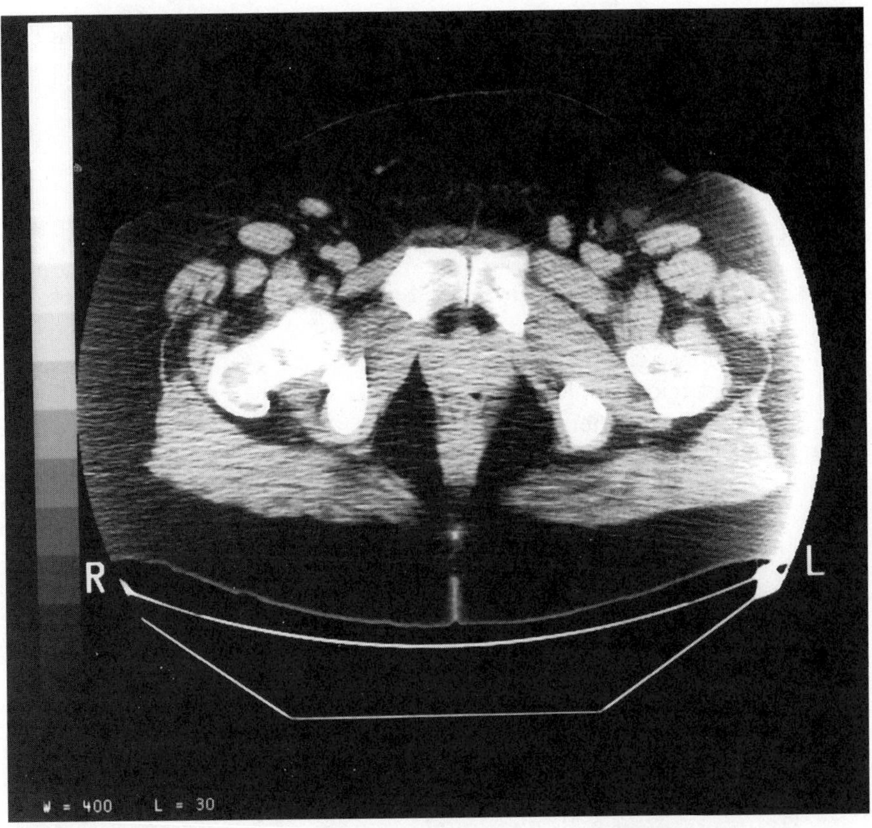

Figure 1–12.

137. The mathematical manipulations required during the reconstruction of a CT image are accomplished using a(n)

1. algorithm
2. kernel
3. mathematical filter function

   a. 1 only
   b. 1 and 2 only
   c. 1 and 3 only
   d. 1, 2, and 3

138. Quality control measurements to test the accuracy of the calibration of the CT scanner should be performed

   a. daily
   b. weekly
   c. monthly
   d. annually

139. Which of the following technical parameters would greatly improve the quality of CT studies requiring multiplanar reformats?

a. noncontiguous scans
b. wide section thicknesses
c. contiguous scans with wide section thickness
d. overlapping scans with narrow section thickness

Questions 140–141 refer to Figure 1–13.

140. The high-density objects labeled as number 2 most likely represent

a. gunshot fragments
b. loose change in patient's clothing
c. surgical staples
d. ingested metallic material

141. Which of the following azimuth settings was used to produce this localizer image?

a. 0°
b. 90°
c. 160°
d. 270°

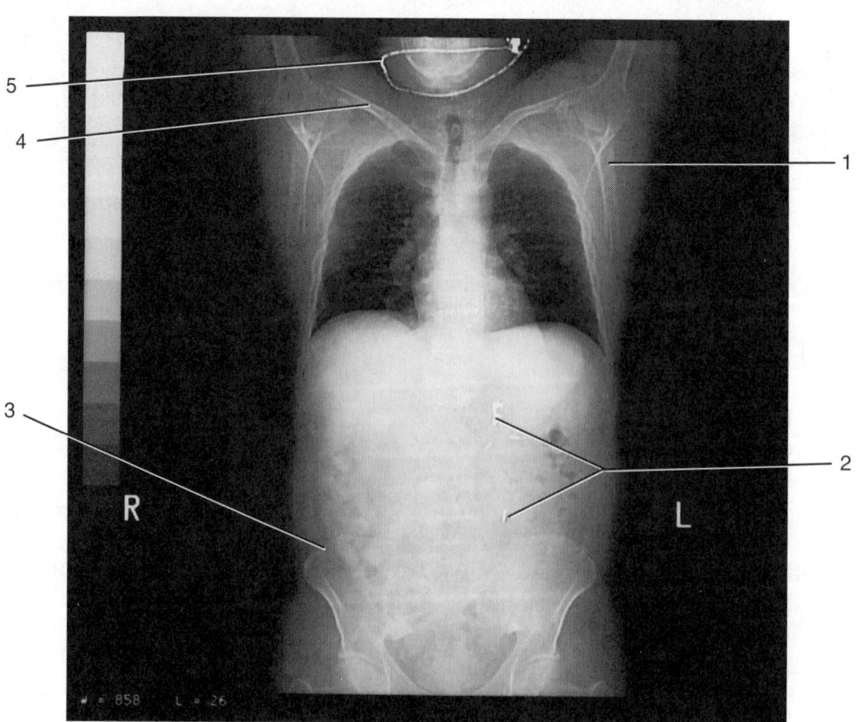

Figure 1–13.

142. Pixels whose average attenuation coefficients are less than that of water have which of the following types of CT number values?

a. extremely large
b. high positive
c. negative
d. none of the above

Question 143 refers to Figure 1–14.

143. Which of the following statements gives the most correct reason why the image of the chest is displayed at a window whose level is −700 and width is 1500?

a. CT images of the lung should always be displayed in predetermined "lung" windows.
b. Soft-tissue demonstration is not required during the CT evaluation of the chest.
c. Strict protocols regarding image display should never be altered by the operator.
d. The level chosen represents the average Hounsfield value for the tissue represented, whereas the width includes the entire range for the anatomy of interest.

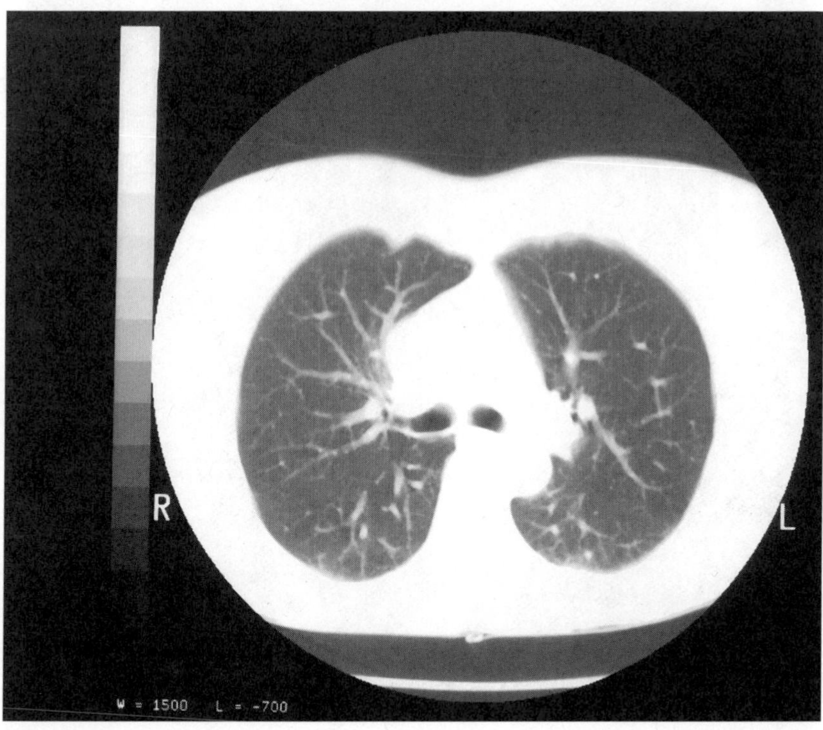

Figure 1–14.

144. Which of the following mathematical techniques is used exclusively for image reconstruction with spiral CT scanners?

a. back-projection
b. convolution
c. interpolation
d. iterative techniques

145. Which of the following reduces scatter radiation reaching the detectors?

a. postpatient collimation
b. prepatient collimation
c. predetector collimation
d. both a and c

146. A voxel may be defined as which of the following?

a. the portion of the CRT displaying the image
b. a miniature image
c. a volume element
d. an arrangement of pixels

Questions 147–148 refer to Figure 1–15.

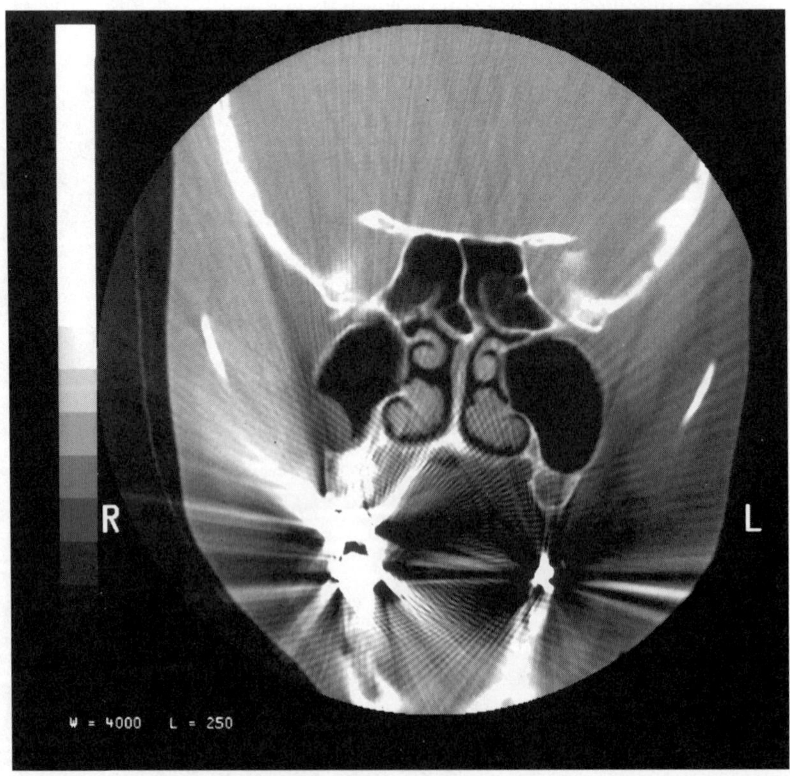

Figure 1–15.

147. Which of the following is the common term for the artifact present on the image?

a. aliasing
b. streaking
c. edge gradient
d. tube arcing

148. Which of the following would be the most common cause of this artifact in this particular case?

a. beam hardening
b. partial volume averaging
c. metallic dental fillings
d. detector malfunction

149. Which of the following would increase spatial resolution of a CT examination using the following parameters: large focal spot size, 10-mm sections, 512- × 512-mm matrix?

1. Change to small focal spot size.
2. Perform 5-mm sections.
3. Reconstruct images in a 320- × 320-mm matrix.

a. 1 only
b. 1 and 2 only
c. 1 and 3 only
d. 1, 2, and 3

150. The portion of the primary beam interacting with a single detector is known as a

a. ray
b. view
c. profile
d. sample

CHAPTER 2

Simulated Exam Two

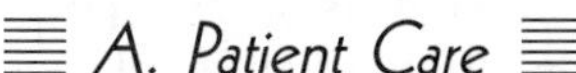

A. Patient Care

1. Which of the following sets of values would be considered normal levels for creatinine and blood urea nitrogen, respectively?

a. 3.1 mg/dL, 1.2 mg/dL
b. 1.2 mg/dL, 14 mg/dL
c. 0.7 mg/dL, 29 mg/dL
d. 5.2 mg/dL, 12 mg/dL

2. Which of the following must be included when obtaining informed consent for an invasive procedure?

1. explanation of the examination techniques
2. the possible risks and benefits of the examination
3. alternatives to the procedure

a. 1 only
b. 1 and 2 only
c. 1 and 3 only
d. 1, 2, and 3

3. Contrast materials that dissociate into charged particles when placed into solution are termed

a. positive
b. non-ionic
c. ionic
d. negative

4. Which of the following is the correct angle of insertion when placing a butterfly needle into a vein for intravenous contrast administration?

a. 5°
b. 15°
c. 45°
d. 60°

5. Which of the following is the correct order for the stages of infection?

a. incubation, prodromal, active, convalescence
b. convalescence, active, prodromal, incubation
c. prodromal, incubation, convalescence, active
d. incubation, convalescence, prodromal, active

6. A normal range for systolic blood pressure in an adult is

a. 40–60 mm Hg
b. 60–90 mm Hg
c. 80–120 mm Hg
d. 95–140 mm Hg

7. After the intrathecal injection of iodinated contrast for a post-myelographic CT study of the lumbar spine, the patient should be instructed to

a. take a cleansing enema
b. resume normal activity
c. rest for 8–24 hours with the head slightly elevated
d. rest for 8–24 hours in the Trendelenburg position

8. The term urticaria is used to describe which of the following?

a. severe nausea with associated vomiting
b. urinary tract infection
c. hives
d. bronchospasm

9. The embryo or fetus is most sensitive to ionizing radiation during which portion of gestation?

a. first trimester
b. second trimester
c. third trimester
d. the fetus is equally radiosensitive during each trimester

10. The rights of the patient include which of the following?

1. The patient has the right to considerate and respectful care.
2. The patient has a right to receive a copy of the diagnostic procedure performed.
3. The patient has the right to refuse medical treatment.

a. 1 only
b. 1 and 2 only
c. 1 and 3 only
d. 1, 2, and 3

11. A patient has a severe vagal reaction to iodinated contrast material that includes bradycardia. Initial treatment may include

a. atropine
b. diazepam
c. ranitidine hydrochloride (Zantac)
d. albuterol sulfate (Proventil)

12. A patient is required to have the following radiographic examinations: CT of the abdomen, gastrointestinal series, and a barium enema. The correct order for the scheduling of these procedures is

a. barium enema, gastrointestinal series, CT of the abdomen
b. gastrointestinal series, CT of the abdomen, barium enema
c. CT of the abdomen, gastrointestinal series, barium enema
d. CT of the abdomen, barium enema, gastrointestinal series

13. The term used to describe the ability of a fluid to flow is

a. density
b. viscosity
c. osmolality
d. specific gravity

14. The normal range of respirations for a child is

a. 5–10 breaths per minute
b. 12–20 breaths per minute
c. 20–30 breaths per minute
d. 35–50 breaths per minute

15. Which of the following drug administration routes provides the most rapid absorption and action within the body?

a. oral
b. subcutaneous
c. intramuscular
d. intravenous

16. The correct order of actions during cardiopulmonary resuscitation is

a. airway, breathing, circulation
b. breathing, airway, circulation
c. airway, circulation, breathing
d. circulation, breathing, airway

17. Where should the tourniquet be positioned when preparing a patient for intravenous contrast administration?

a. directly over the injection site
b. proximal to the injection site
c. distal to the injection site
d. below the injection site

18. Iodine is a common material used in radiopaque contrast media due to its

a. radiolucency
b. viscosity
c. osmolality
d. high atomic number

19. Examples of severe adverse reactions to iodinated intravenous contrast media may include

1. anaphylaxis
2. urticaria
3. vomiting

a. 1 only
b. 1 and 2 only
c. 1 and 3 only
d. 1, 2, and 3

20. Which of the following statements is true concerning site preparation with an antiseptic for an invasive procedure?

a. The area should be dabbed with an antiseptic-moistened paper towel.
b. The area should be painted with antiseptic in a linear motion.
c. The area should be painted with antiseptic in a circular motion, beginning at the center and working outward.
d. The area should be painted with antiseptic in a circular motion, beginning at the outer margins and working inward.

21. Which of the following interactions between x-ray and matter results in the largest amount of occupational exposure?

a. characteristic effect
b. Compton effect
c. bremsstrahlung effect
d. photoelectric effect

22. Which of the following should be included as instructions to the patient before beginning any CT examination?

a. The examination to be performed—for example, what area of the body is to be studied—should be described.
b. The process of contrast administration should be explained.
c. Any necessary breathing instructions should be given clearly and precisely.
d. All of the above apply.

23. A high osmolar contrast material has an average osmolality of

a. 100–300 mOsm/kg water
b. 600–850 mOsm/kg water
c. 1000–2400 mOsm/kg water
d. 4000–7000 mOsm/kg water

24. Which of the following sets of injection flow rates is a biphasic technique for a spiral CT study of the liver?

a. 2 mL/sec for 100 mL with scanning during both peak enhancement and the equilibrium phase
b. 3 mL/sec for 150 mL with a 90-second delay before scanning
c. 2 mL/sec for 50 mL during the superior half of the liver
d. 3 mL/sec for 50 mL followed by 1.5 mL/sec for 100 mL

25. Infection may occur indirectly through contact with contaminated objects known as

a. vectors
b. fomites
c. vehicles
d. hosts

26. Which of the following terms is used to describe a patient having difficulty swallowing?

a. dyslexia
b. dyspnea
c. dysphagia
d. dysphasia

27. The normal platelet count range for an adult is

a. 30,000–45,000/mm^3 of blood
b. 75,000–125,000/mm^3 of blood
c. 150,000–400,000/mm^3 of blood
d. 450,000–700,000/mm^3 of blood

28. Intravenous contrast administration with an automatic injector during a CT examination is usually performed through

a. Infuse-A-Ports
b. angiocatheters
c. port-A-Caths
d. Hickman catheters

29. Late effects of radiation such as genetic mutations may occur with even small doses of radiation and are termed

a. stochastic
b. somatic
c. nonstochastic
d. chronic

30. The choice of ionic versus non-ionic contrast administration should be based on

1. the allergic history of the patient
2. the cost of the contrast material
3. the age and physical condition of the patient

a. 1 only
b. 1 and 2 only
c. 1 and 3 only
d. 1, 2, and 3

B. Imaging Procedures

31. The abdominal aorta bifurcates at the level of

a. T10
b. T12
c. L2
d. L4

32. Quantitative CT is a specialized technique used most often for the diagnosis of

a. lymphoma
b. osteoporosis
c. renal cyst
d. hemangioma

Questions 33–36 refer to Figure 2–1.

33. Which of the following algorithms was used in the reconstruction of the image?

a. bone
b. edge
c. soft tissue
d. detail

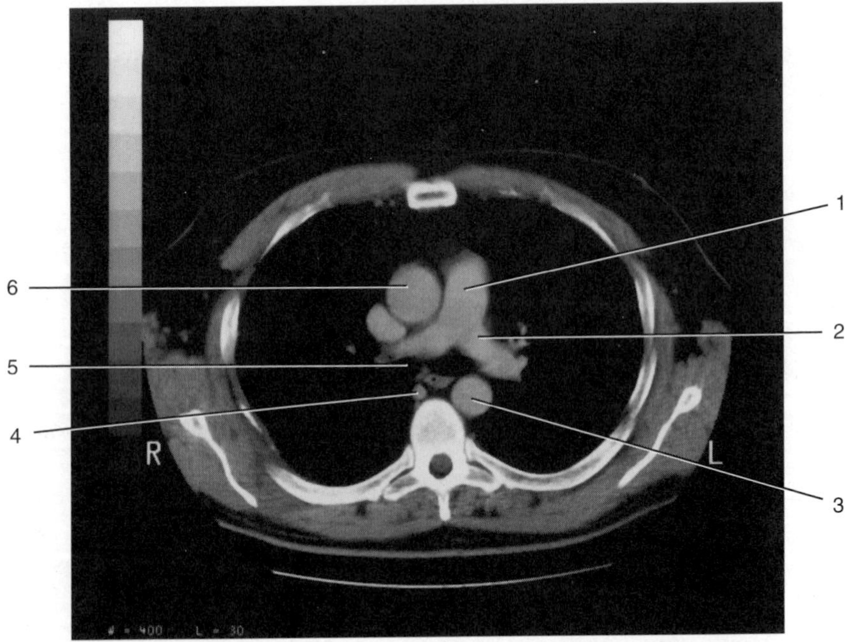

Figure 2–1.

34. Number 2 corresponds to which of the following?

a. left primary bronchus
b. descending aorta
c. superior vena cava
d. left pulmonary artery

35. Which number corresponds to the right primary bronchus?

a. 6
b. 3
c. 5
d. 1

36. Number 3 corresponds to which of the following?

a. descending aorta
b. inferior vena cava
c. left pulmonary artery
d. esophagus

37. The average density of a mass within the kidney measures −75 Hounsfield units. This mass is most likely a

a. cyst
b. lipoma
c. stone
d. hydrocele

38. Which of the following is a common complication during CT-guided biopsy of the lung?

a. pulmonary embolism
b. aspiration
c. pneumoconiosis
d. pneumothorax

Questions 39–43 refer to Figure 2–2.

39. Number 4 corresponds to which of the following?

a. cochlea

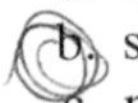

b. semicircular canal

c. malleus

d. incus

40. Number 5 corresponds to which of the following?

a. dorsum sella

b. anterior clinoid process

c. petrous bone

d. posterior clinoid process

41. Which of the following window level and width settings was used to display the image?

a. L = −700, W = 2000

b. L = +50, W = 400

c. L = +150, W = 1000

d. L = +250, W = 4000

42. Number 1 corresponds to which of the following?

a. dorsum sella

b. sphenoid sinus

c. ethmoid sinus

d. pituitary fossa

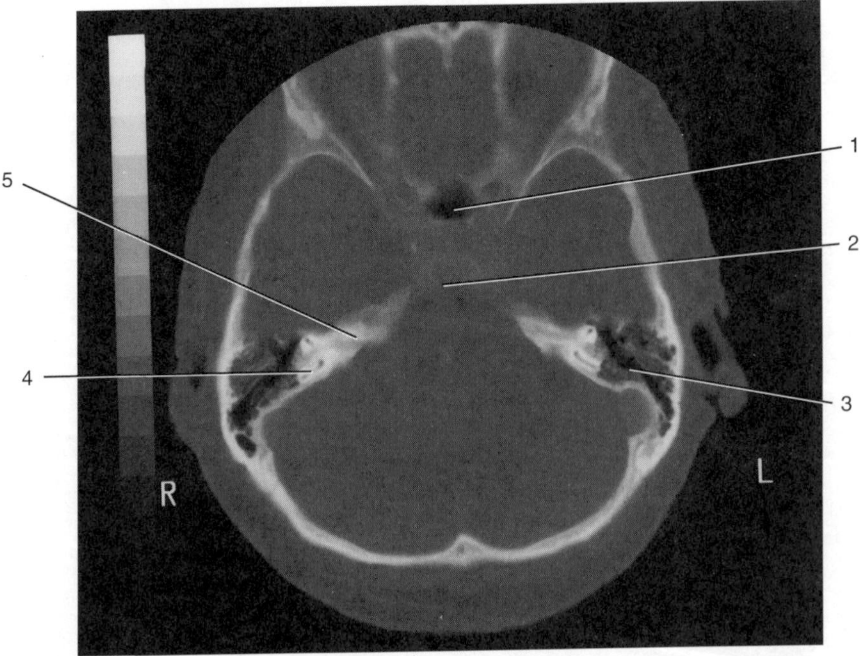

Figure 2–2.

43. Which of the following is the best choice for scan field of view (SFOV) for the acquisition of the image?

a. small (25 cm)
b. head (25 cm)
c. medium (35 cm)
d. large (48 cm)

44. CT images of the abdomen should be acquired with the patient

a. at full inspiration
b. breathing quietly
c. at full expiration
d. breathing normally

45. Which of the following types of contrast material may be used during CT evaluation of the pelvis?

1. intravenous iodinated contrast
2. low-density barium sulfate solutions
3. oil-based contrast material

a. 1 only
b. 2 only
c. 1 and 2 only
d. 1, 2, and 3

Questions 46–48 refer to Figure 2–3.

46. Which number corresponds to the common carotid artery?

a. 4
b. 3
c. 1
d. 5

47. Number 4 corresponds to which of the following?

a. internal jugular vein
b. external carotid artery
c. internal carotid artery
d. retromandibular vein

48. Number 2 corresponds to which of the following?

a. trapezius muscle
b. levator scapulae muscle
c. sternocleidomastoid muscle
d. parotid gland

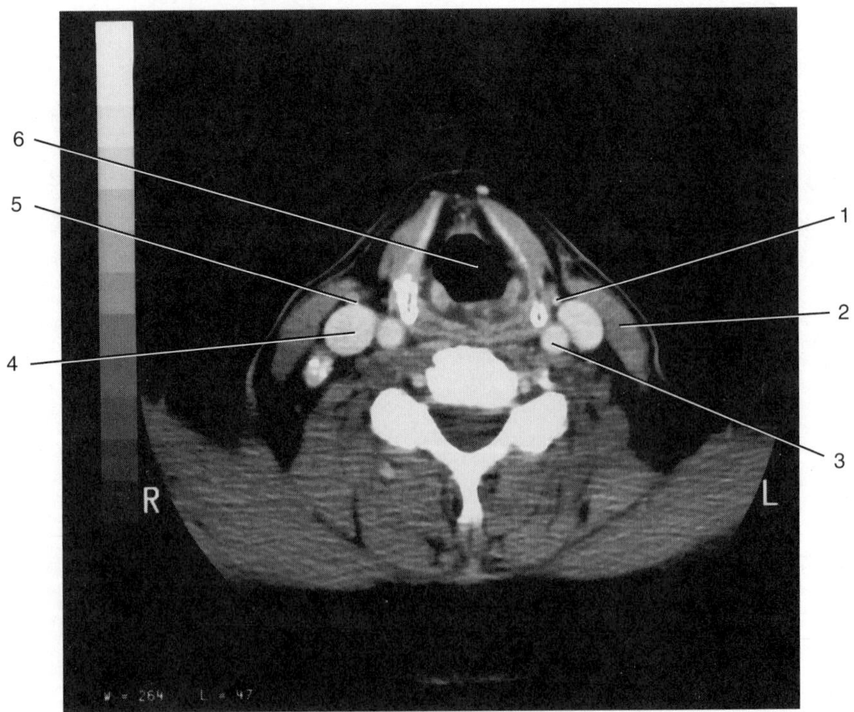

Figure 2–3.

49. Which of the following would be a suitable range for contrast volume for an intrathecal injection during a post-myelogram CT examination of the lumbar spine in an adult patient?

a. 1–3 mL
b. 5–9 mL
c. 12–14 mL
d. 18–22 mL

50. Of the following ranges, which would be most suited for a scout (localizer) image of the abdomen?

a. below the diaphragm to the bottom of the kidneys
b. top of the kidneys to the level of the midsacrum
c. top of the kidneys to the umbilicus
d. above the diaphragm to the iliac crest

Questions 51–53 refer to Figure 2–4.

51. Number 4 corresponds to which of the following?
   a. lateral condyle
   b. medial condyle
   c. lateral epicondyle
   d. medial epicondyle

52. Number 3 corresponds to which of the following?
   a. retropatellar space
   b. medial meniscus
   c. tibial collateral ligament
   d. intercondylar fossa

53. During this CT examination of the knee, the patient was most likely in the ______________ position.
   a. ventral recumbent
   b. right lateral
   c. supine
   d. left lateral

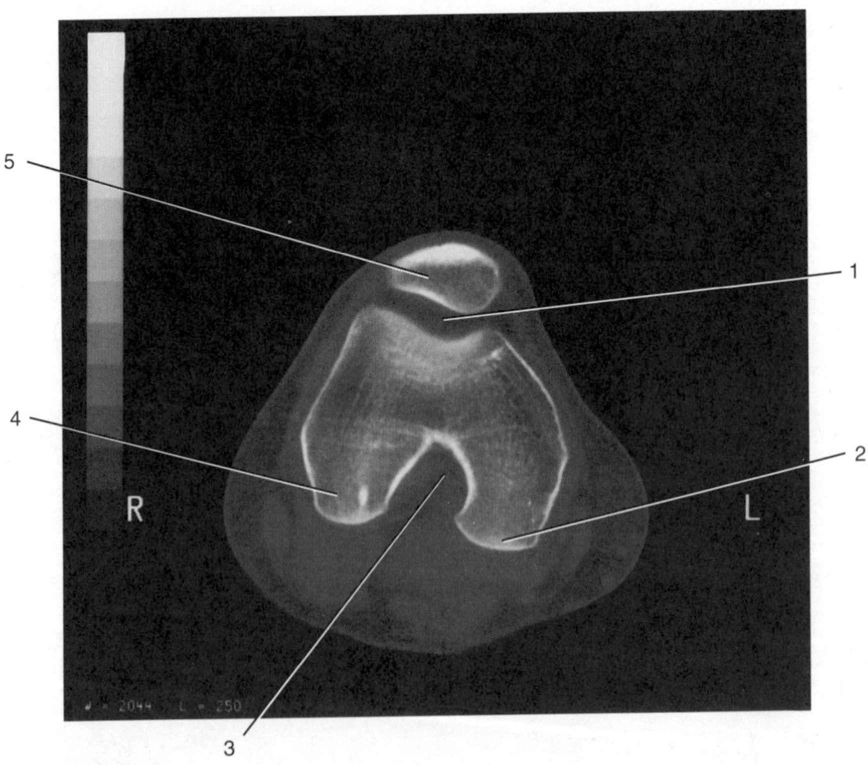

Figure 2–4.

54. To reduce peristalsis and distend the colon, ______________ may be administered before a CT scan of the abdomen or pelvis.

a. diazepam (Valium)
b. glucagon
c. prochlorperazine maleate (Compazine)
d. bisacodyl (Dulcolax)

55. A common, nonmalignant enlargement of the prostate gland is typically referred to as

a. prostatic carcinoma
b. prostatic abscess
c. prostatic hypertrophy
d. extraprostatic extension

Questions 56–59 refer to Figure 2–5.

56. Number 2 corresponds to which of the following?
   a. right brachiocephalic vein
   b. left subclavian artery
   c. left brachiocephalic vein
   d. brachiocephalic artery

57. Number 5 corresponds to which of the following?
   a. right brachiocephalic vein
   b. left subclavian artery
   c. left brachiocephalic vein
   d. brachiocephalic artery

58. Number 1 corresponds to which of the following?
   a. right brachiocephalic vein
   b. left subclavian artery
   c. left brachiocephalic vein
   d. brachiocephalic artery

59. Which number corresponds to the left common carotid artery?
   a. 1
   b. 6
   c. 4
   d. 3

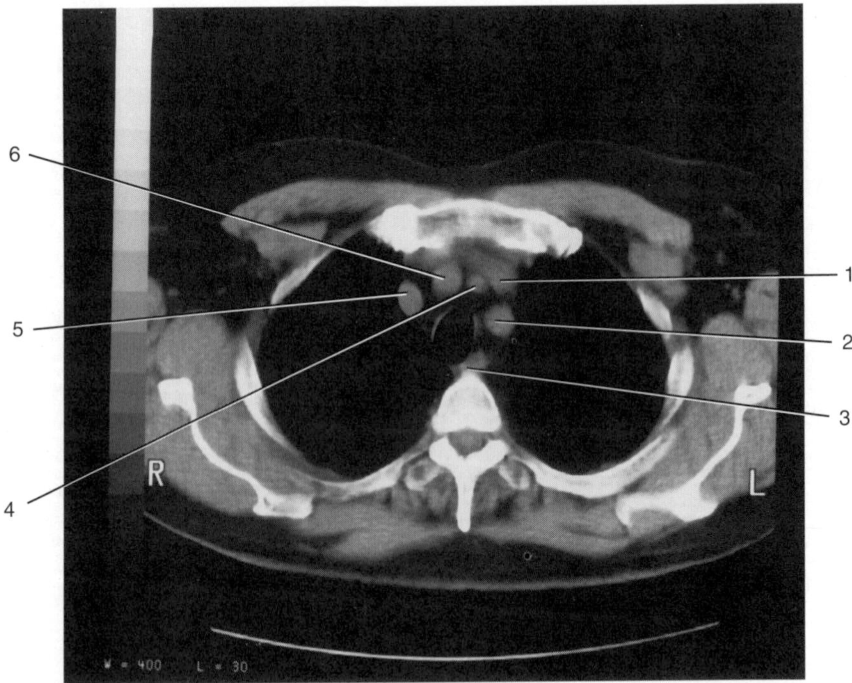

Figure 2–5.

60. After the intravenous administration of iodinated contrast media, a hepatic hemangioma may become ______________ and no longer appear on the CT image.

a. hypodense
b. radiolucent
c. isodense
d. hyperdense

61. Which of the following are advantages of spiral or helical CT over conventional CT scanning?

1. reduced scan time
2. reduction of misregistration artifacts
3. decreased patient dose

a. 1 only
b. 1 and 2 only
c. 1 and 3 only
d. 1, 2, and 3

Questions 62–65 refer to Figure 2–6.

62. Number 5 corresponds to which of the following?
- a. transverse colon
- b. stomach
- c. duodenum
- d. hepatic flexure

63. Which of the following most likely describes the patient position?
- a. supine
- b. prone
- c. left lateral decubitus
- d. right lateral decubitus

64. CT examinations of the abdomen are often performed in this position to demonstrate the relationship between the
- a. ureters and renal collecting systems
- b. duodenum and pancreatic head
- c. large and small colon
- d. liver and gallbladder

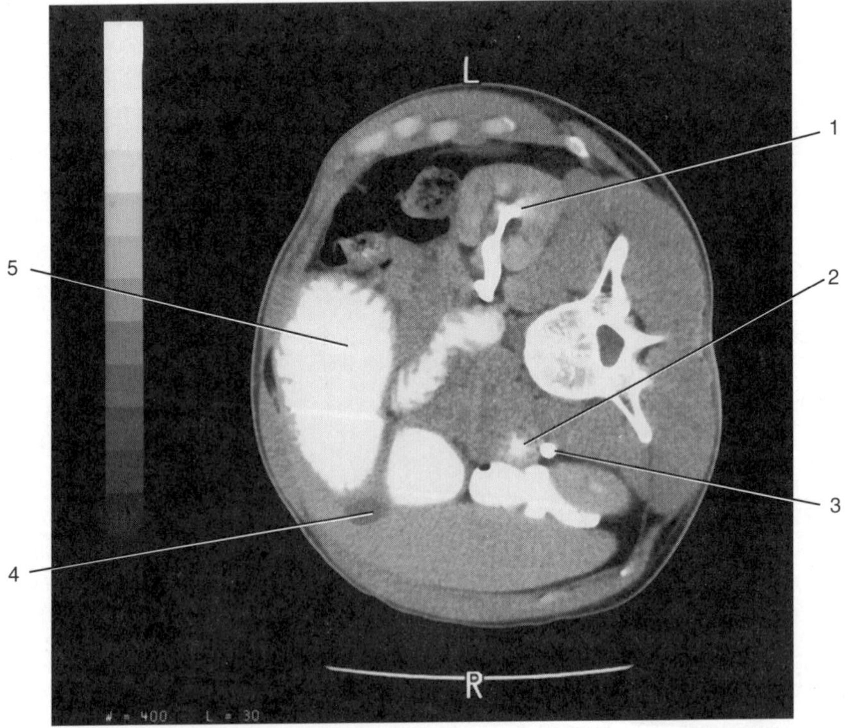

Figure 2–6.

65. Number 3 corresponds to which of the following?

a. right ureter
b. inferior vena cava
c. renal calculi
d. right renal artery

66. Which of the following areas of the head commonly become calcified?

1. thalamus
2. pineal gland
3. choroid plexus

a. 2 only
b. 1 and 3 only
c. 2 and 3 only
d. 1, 2, and 3

67. Owing to its excessive density, barium sulfate may be used in CT examinations only in suspensions with concentrations of

a. 1%–3% barium sulfate
b. 5%–7% barium sulfate
c. 10%–13% barium sulfate
d. 25%–30% barium sulfate

Questions 68–70 refer to Figure 2–7.

68. Number 4 corresponds to which of the following?

a. pedicle
b. spinous process
c. lamina
d. transverse process

69. Number 6 corresponds to which of the following?

a. anterior process
b. lamina
c. body
d. superior articulating process

70. Which number corresponds to the foramen transversarium?

a. 5
b. 3
c. 1
d. 2

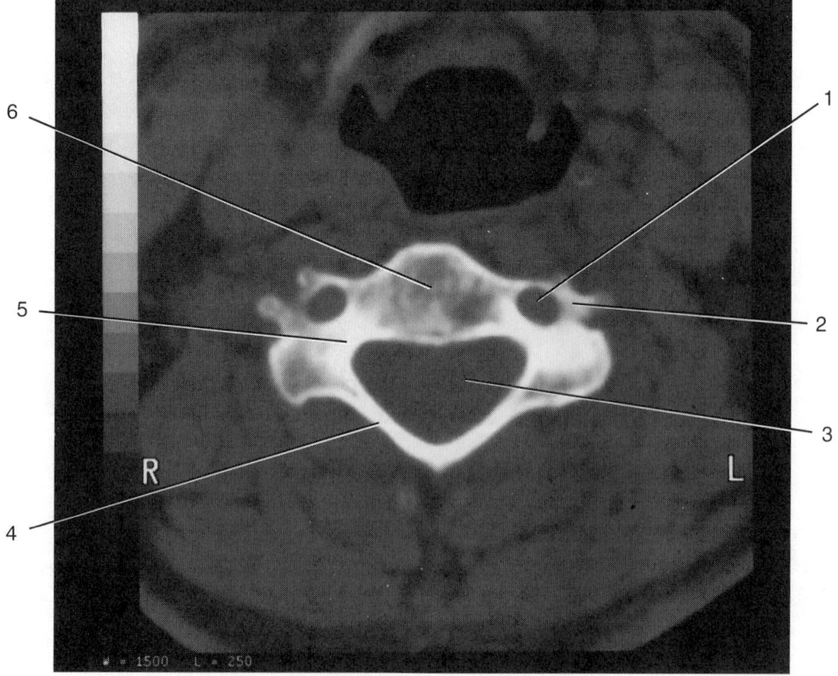

Figure 2–7.

71. Accurate demonstration of ______________ would most likely require the intravenous injection of iodinated contrast during a CT study of the abdomen.

a. appendicitis
b. a renal stone
c. diverticulitis
d. a renal cyst

72. During CT scanning of the head, the gantry should be angled

a. 15° above the orbitomeatal line
b. 10° below the infraorbitomeatal line
c. 0°
d. 20° above the skull base

73. Which of the following types of CT scanners is best suited for the evaluation of coronary artery disease?

a. spiral
b. fourth generation
c. ultrafast
d. third generation

Questions 74–77 refer to Figure 2–8.

74. Considering only the image, which of the following types of contrast material were administered to the patient?

1. oral
2. intravenous
3. rectal

a. 1 only
b. 2 only
c. 1 and 2 only
d. 1, 2, and 3

75. Number 3 corresponds to which of the following?

a. seminal vesicles
b. rectal tendon
c. anus
d. ureters

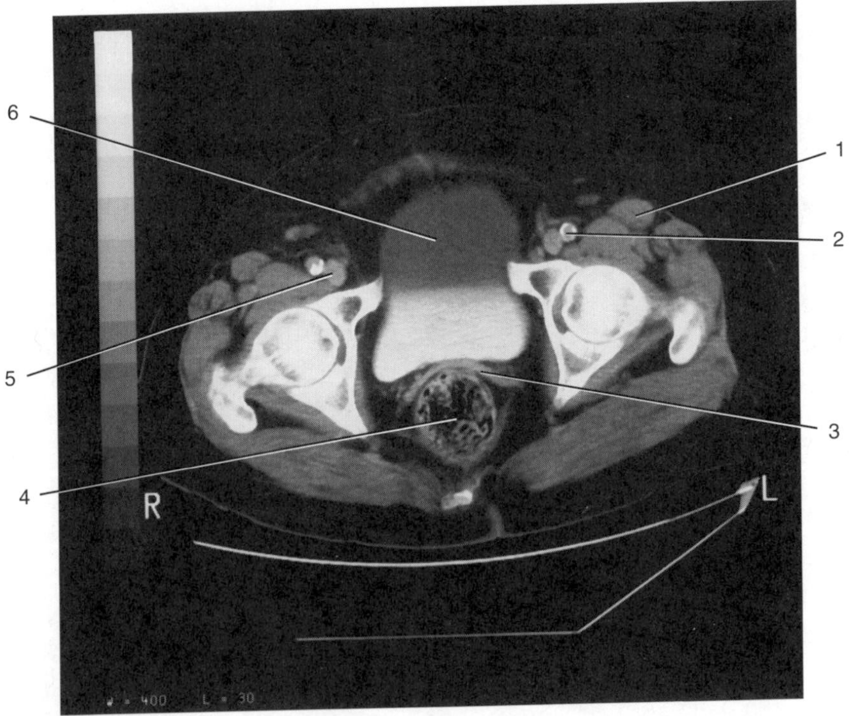

Figure 2–8.

76. Number 2 corresponds to which of the following?

a. iliac artery
b. femoral vein
c. iliac vein
d. femoral artery

77. Number 1 corresponds to which of the following?

a. iliopsoas muscle
b. sartorius muscle
c. gluteus minimus muscle
d. rectus femoris muscle

78. High-resolution CT of the chest incorporates which of the following protocols?

a. 10-mm sections, standard algorithm
b. 10-mm sections, bone algorithm
c. 3-mm sections, standard algorithm
d. 1-mm sections, bone algorithm

79. Dynamic CT scanning involves which of the following technical considerations?

1. data acquisition with the patient continuously moving through the gantry
2. bolus administration of iodinated intravenous contrast media
3. rapid scanning with minimal interscan delays

a. 1 only
b. 1 and 3 only
c. 2 and 3 only
d. 1, 2, and 3

80. Which of the following terms describes the appearance of an acute subdural hematoma on a CT image of the brain?

a. radiolucent
b. hyperdense
c. hypodense
d. isodense

Questions 81–85 refer to Figure 2–9.

81. Number 4 corresponds to which of the following?

a. iliac crest
b. anterior superior iliac spine
c. anterior inferior iliac spine
d. posterior inferior iliac spine

82. Which of the following best describes the position of the patient?

a. prone with hands behind back
b. ventral recumbent with hands over head
c. dorsal recumbent with hands above head
d. supine with hands crossed over chest

83. Number 1 corresponds to which of the following?

a. ascending colon
b. hepatic flexure
c. splenic flexure
d. transverse colon

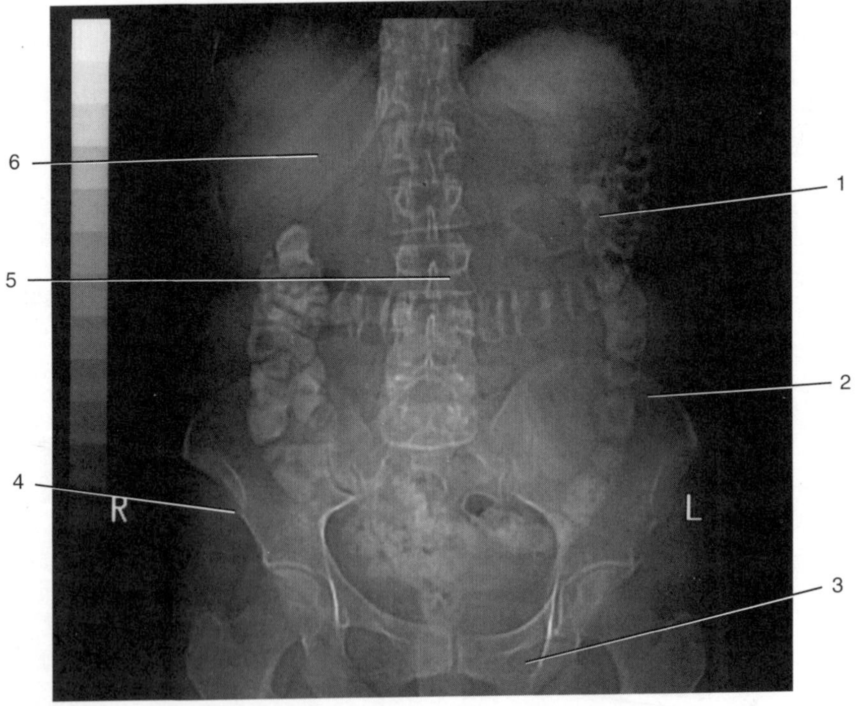

Figure 2–9.

84. The localizer (scanogram) image could be used to program which of the following CT examinations?

1. abdomen only
2. chest and abdomen
3. abdomen and pelvis
   a. 1 only
   b. 1 and 2 only
   c. 1 and 3 only
   d. 1, 2, and 3

85. Number 3 corresponds to which of the following?

a. pelvic outlet
b. pubic arch
c. greater sciatic notch
d. obturator foramen

86. Positioning the patient with the knees flexed over a foam cushion during a CT examination of the lumbar spine assists in

1. decreasing the kyphotic curvature of the lumbar spine
2. making the patient more comfortable throughout the examination
3. decreasing the lordotic curvature of the lumbar spine
   a. 1 only
   b. 2 only
   c. 3 only
   d. 2 and 3 only

87. Which of the following would not be considered an absolute contraindication to intravenous iodinated contrast during CT examination of the kidneys?

a. pheochromocytoma
b. acute sickle cell anemia
c. allergies to shellfish
d. prior major reaction to contrast media

88. A solitary pulmonary nodule can be assumed to be benign when its average density is within which of the following ranges?

a. 10–30 Hounsfield units
b. 45–80 Hounsfield units
c. 100–140 Hounsfield units
d. 165–200 Hounsfield units

Questions 89–91 refer to Figure 2–10.

89. Number 5 corresponds to which of the following?
- a. femoral head
- b. coracoid process
- c. acromion
- d. humeral head

90. Number 2 corresponds to which of the following?
- a. acromion
- b. glenoid fossa
- c. coronoid process
- d. acetabulum

91. The multiplanar reconstruction image was formed from CT images using which of the following sets of section widths and spacing?
- a. 3 × 3 mm
- b. 5 × 10 mm
- c. 10 × 10 mm
- d. 10 × 12 mm

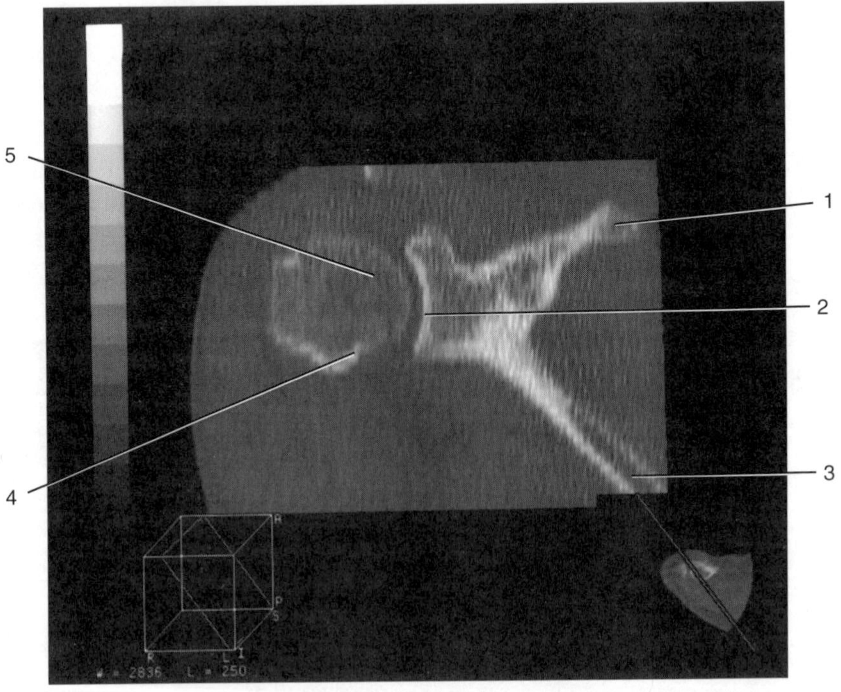

Figure 2–10.

92. After the injection of intravenous contrast media during a CT examination of the brain, which of the following anatomic areas does not enhance?

a. anterior communicating artery
b. choroid plexus
c. posterior horn of lateral ventricle
d. dura mater

93. Which of the following techniques assists in visualizing the vagina during a CT study of the pelvis?

a. tampon insertion
b. precontrast and postcontrast scanning
c. oral contrast administration
d. enema contrast administration

Questions 94–97 refer to Figure 2–11.

94. Number 2 corresponds to which of the following?
   a. splenic vein
   b. left renal artery
   c. pancreas
   d. duodenum

95. Which of the following methods of oral contrast administration is suitable for the CT scan of the abdomen depicted in the figure?
   a. 1500 mL, 90–120 minutes before scanning
   b. 1200-mL enema immediately before scanning
   c. 100 mL, 6 hours before scanning, with an additional 50 mL given just before the study
   d. 500 mL, 30 minutes before scanning, with an additional 300 mL given just before the study

96. Number 3 corresponds to which of the following?
   a. inferior mesenteric artery
   b. adrenal gland
   c. tail of pancreas
   d. renal vein

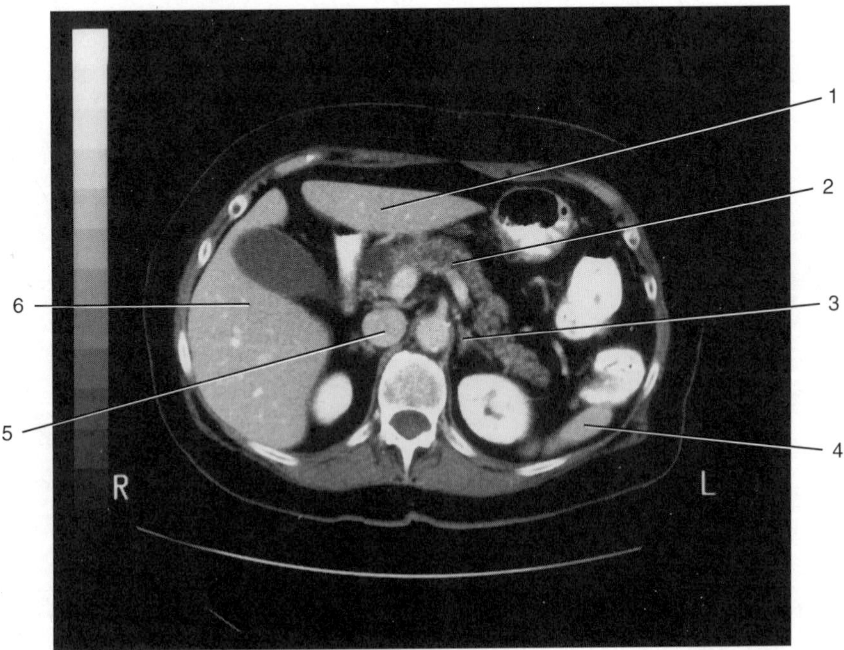

Figure 2–11.

97. Which number corresponds to the left lobe of the liver?

a. 5
b. 1
c. 4
d. 6

98. The plane that passes vertically through the body, dividing it into left and right portions, is referred to as the

a. orthogonal plane
b. axial plane
c. sagittal plane
d. coronal plane

99. Which of the following are reasons for intravenous contrast to be administered during CT evaluation of the pelvis?

1. distension and contrast enhancement of the bladder
2. visualization of the rectosigmoid junction
3. differentiation of blood vessels and pelvic lymph nodes

a. 1 only
b. 1 and 2 only
c. 1 and 3 only
d. 1, 2, and 3

Questions 100–103 refer to Figure 2–12.

100. Number 1 corresponds to which of the following?
- a. splenium of corpus callosum
- b. internal capsule
- c. body of corpus callosum
- d. genu of corpus callosum

101. Number 6 corresponds to which of the following?
- a. anterior cerebral artery
- b. falx cerebri
- c. callosal marginal artery
- d. middle cerebral artery

102. Which number corresponds to the internal capsule?
- a. 1
- b. 2
- c. 4
- d. 6

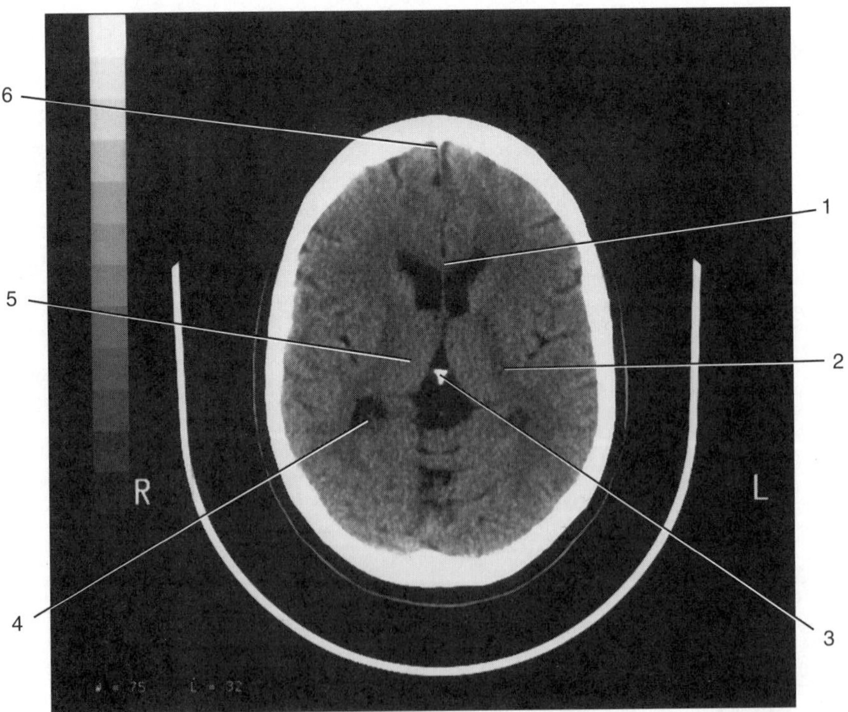

Figure 2–12.

103. Number 3 corresponds to which of the following?

a. pineal gland
b. middle cerebral artery
c. fourth ventricle
d. aqueduct of Sylvius

104. Which of the following display fields of view (DFOVs) should be chosen for a CT examination of the thoracic spine of a patient whose thorax measures 40 cm?

a. 15 cm
b. 25 cm
c. 32 cm
d. 42 cm

105. The presence of outpocketings in the wall of the colon is referred to as

a. intussusception
b. diverticulitis
c. polyps
d. diverticulosis

C. Physics and Instrumentation

106. Which of the following is the Lambert-Beer law that describes the relationship between matter and attenuation?

a. Attenuation = I_0/I
b. CT number = $\dfrac{\mu_t - \mu_w}{\mu_w} \times K$
c. $I_0 = Ix^{e\mu}$
d. $I = I_0e^{-\mu x}$

107. A pixel may be defined as

a. the portion of the CRT displaying the image
b. a volume element
c. a picture element
d. a miniature image

108. The mathematical technique that involves the estimation of an unknown value from values on either side of it is known as

a. filtering
b. interpolation
c. convolution
d. summation

109. Pixels representing tissues with average attenuation coefficients greater than that of water have which of the following types of values?

a. extremely small
b. positive
c. negative
d. none of the above

110. When compared with conventional radiography, CT produces diagnostic images with improved

a. low-contrast resolution
b. spatial resolution
c. minute detail
d. patient dose reduction

111. In 1917, the Austrian mathematician ______________ proved that it was possible to reconstruct a three-dimensional object from the infinite set of all of its projections.

a. Radon
b. Tsien
c. Bracewell
d. Cormack

112. Which of the following is not commonly used as a CT scintillation detector material?

a. ceramic rare earth
b. silver halide
c. bismuth germinate
d. cadmium tungstate

Questions 113–115 refer to Figure 2–13.

113. The region of interest measurement in the figure provides an average density of +1.9 Hounsfield units. This material is most likely
   a. fat
   b. blood
   c. tumor
   d. water

114. The material within the region of interest measurement has a linear attenuation coefficient of approximately
   a. 0.0007
   b. 0.155
   c. 0.206
   d. 0.530

115. The image was displayed using which of the following window widths?
   a. 70
   b. 400
   c. 1300
   d. 3800

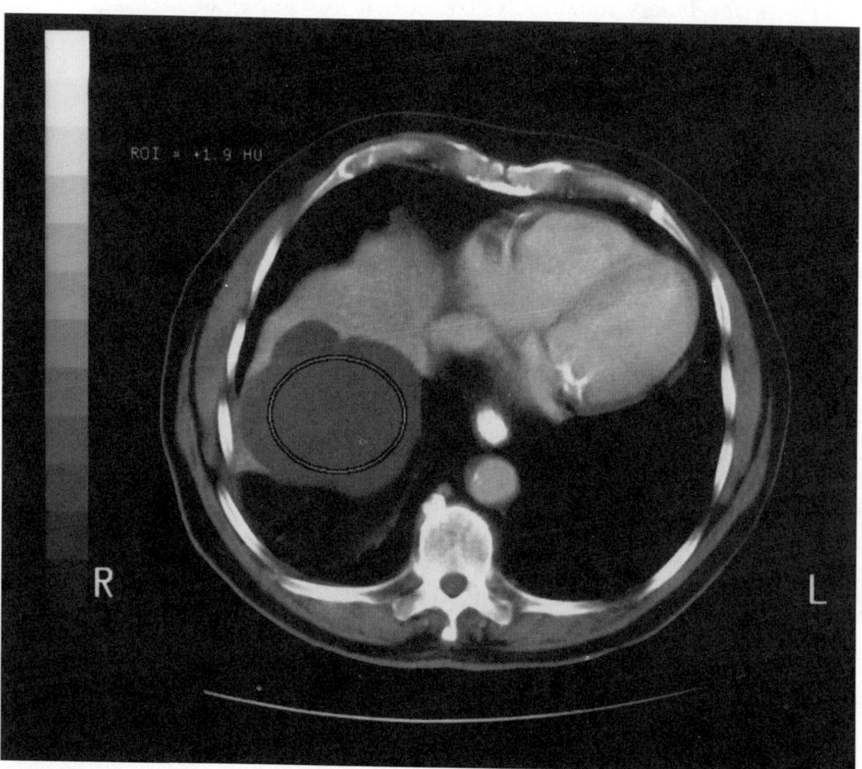

Figure 2–13.

116. Which of the following is the primary interaction between x-ray photons and tissue during CT examination?

a. bremsstrahlung effect
b. characteristic effect
c. Compton effect
d. coherent scatter

117. Areas of a CT image that contain minimal changes in tissue density are electronically represented by

a. positive CT numbers
b. high spatial frequencies
c. negative CT numbers
d. low spatial frequencies

118. Ring artifacts on the CT image are associated with which of the following tube–detector geometric relationships?

a. rotate–nutate
b. rotate–stationary
c. rotate–rotate
d. translate–rotate

119. In the binary number system, a byte is a series of __________ bits of information.

a. 2
b. 4
c. 8
d. 16

120. An accurate, modern CT scanner is capable of a spatial resolution of up to

a. 10 lp/mm
b. 20 lp/mm
c. 10 lp/cm
d. 20 lp/cm

121. Which of the following is the best method to reduce respiratory motion on the CT image?

a. good patient–technologist communication
b. reduced scan times
c. use of immobilization devices
d. glucagon administration

122. Which of the following statements is correct regarding the radiographic film used to archive CT images?

1. It is a double-emulsion film.
2. It is sensitive to ultraviolet light only.
3. It may be used in conjunction with a multiformat or laser camera.

a. 1 only
b. 2 only
c. 3 only
d. 1 and 3 only

123. Which of the following reconstruction methods is used by most modern CT scanners?
  a. back-projection
  b. iterative methods
  c. Fourier transform
  d. filtered back-projection

124. Fourth-generation CT scanners use a ____________ tube–detector configuration.
  a. rotate–translate
  b. electron beam–stationary
  c. rotate–stationary
  d. rotate–rotate

125. The fluctuation of CT numbers in an image of uniform, homogeneous material is known as
  a. linearity
  b. noise
  c. artifact
  d. partial volume effect

126. The term "beam hardening" describes which of the following physical phenomena?
  a. the decrease in average photon energy of a heterogeneous x-ray beam
  b. the increase in average photon energy of a homogeneous x-ray beam
  c. the increase in average photon energy of a heterogeneous x-ray beam
  d. none of the above

127. The process by which electrons are produced at the cathode of a CT x-ray tube is known as
  a. rectification
  b. anode heel effect
  c. thermionic emission
  d. isotropic emission

128. Which of the following increases the signal-to-noise ratio of a CT image?
  a. decreased aperture size
  b. decreased milliampere-seconds (mAs)
  c. increased filtration
  d. increased aperture size

129. A straight line appearing vertically on the scanogram (pilot) of a fourth-generation CT scanner is an artifact most likely caused by
  a. edge gradient
  b. detector malfunction
  c. tube arcing
  d. beam hardening

130. The acronym CTDI is used to describe which of the following?

a. a specialized CT imaging technique used to measure bone mineral density
b. a quality control test that measures the accuracy of the laser lighting system
c. the radiation dose to the patient during a CT scan
d. a high-speed CT scanner used for cardiac imaging

131. What is the DFOV used for a 320^2 matrix image with a pixel dimension of .75 × .75 mm?

a. 12 cm
b. 24 cm
c. 36 cm
d. 48 cm

132. The full width at half-maximum of a CT scanner is used to describe

a. spatial resolution
b. contrast resolution
c. noise
d. calibration accuracy

133. The average photon energy of the primary beam of a CT scanner operating at a tube potential of 120 kVp is

a. 50 keV
b. 70 keV
c. 100 keV
d. 120 keV

Questions 134–136 refer to Figure 2–14.

134. The image artifact shown in the figure is commonly referred to as

a. partial volume effect
b. motion artifact
c. edge gradient effect
d. ring artifact

135. Which of the following would reduce the image artifact shown?

1. increase filtration
2. increase kVp
3. increase aperture size

a. 1 only
b. 1 and 2 only
c. 1 and 3 only
d. 1, 2, and 3

136. The image was most likely displayed in a window with a level of

a. −150
b. 0
c. +50
d. +400

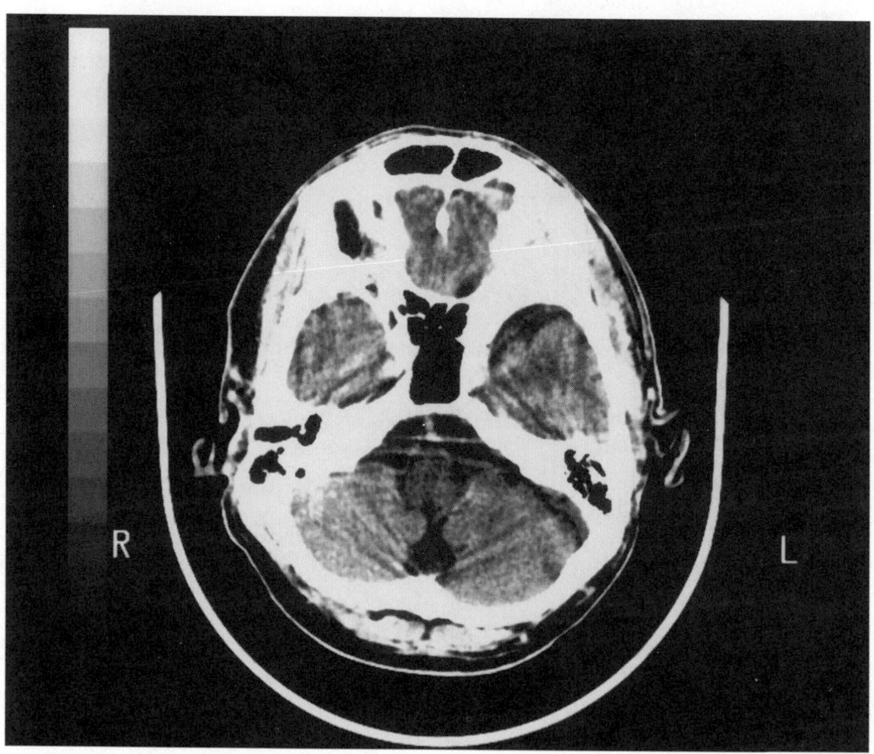

Figure 2–14.

137. Which of the following is not a typical matrix size used with a modern CT scanner?

a. 80 × 80
b. 320 × 320
c. 512 × 512
d. 1024 × 1024

138. Which of the following statements regarding collimation of the CT x-ray beam is false?

a. Collimation of the x-ray beam occurs both before and after the beam passes through the patient.
b. Collimation of the beam occurs in the z-axis, thus controlling slice thickness.
c. Increases in collimation increase the intensity of the primary beam.
d. Collimation of the CT x-ray beam is used to limit the detection of scatter radiation.

139. Statistical noise appears as ________________ on a CT image.

a. decreased contrast
b. increased brightness
c. concentric circles
d. graininess

140. A quality control procedure determines that the low-contrast resolution of a CT scanner is extremely poor. Causes may include

1. increased tube output
2. increased electronic noise
3. decreased patient dose

a. 1 only
b. 1 and 3 only
c. 2 and 3 only
d. 1, 2, and 3

141. Where is the high-frequency generator usually located in a modern CT scanner?

a. inside the gantry
b. just outside the scan room
c. beneath the CT table
d. inside the operator's console

142. The information included during the three-dimensional reconstruction of a CT scan is controlled by the

a. algorithm
b. window setting
c. threshold setting
d. gray scale map

143. Which of the following components of CT image quality may be controlled by the technologist?

1. spatial resolution
2. contrast resolution
3. noise
   a. 2 only
   b. 3 only
   c. 1 and 3 only
   d. 1, 2, and 3

144. The device constructed to house the x-ray tube and data acquisition system for a CT scanner is termed the

a. central processing unit
b. generator
c. array processor
d. gantry

145. Partial volume averaging occurs within a renal cyst during a spiral CT scan of the abdomen. Which of the following technical adjustments could reduce the partial volume effect and provide more accurate CT numbers?

1. retrospective reconstruction of the scan using a reduced section thickness
2. rescanning of the patient using a reduced section thickness
3. retrospective reconstruction of the scan using a reduced section spacing
   a. 2 only
   b. 1 and 2 only
   c. 2 and 3 only
   d. 1, 2, and 3

146. A 512 × 512 matrix consists of how many pixels?

a. 512
b. 1024
c. 26,214
d. 262,144

Question 147 refers to Figure 2–15.

147. The artifact present in the figure was most likely caused by

a. patient motion
b. surgical staples
c. gallstones
d. detector malfunction

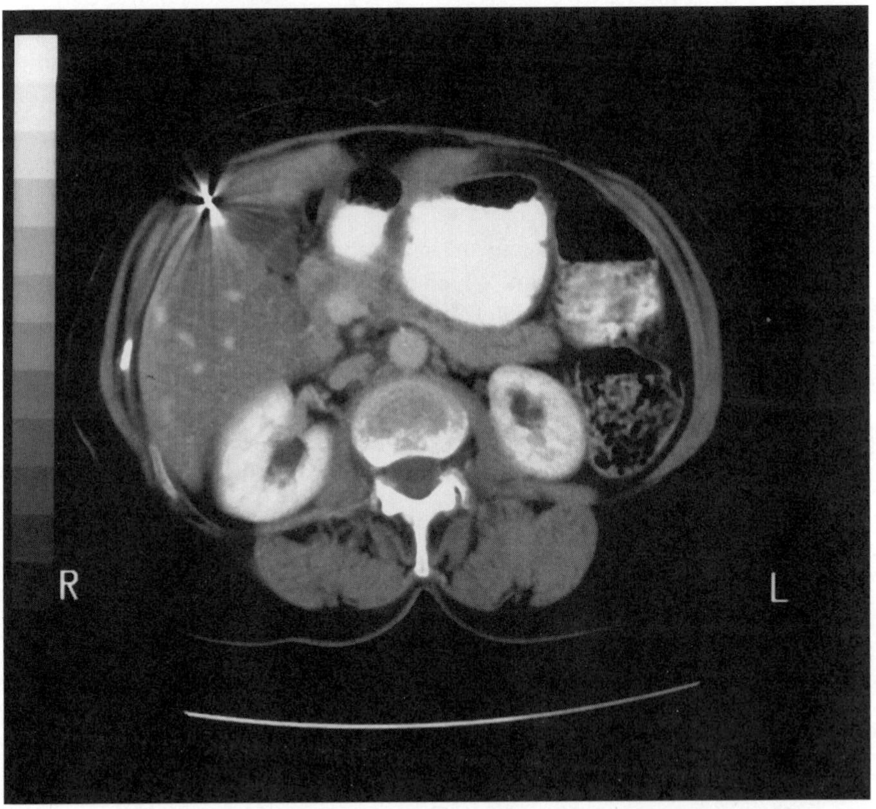

Figure 2–15.

148. The Hounsfield value of a pixel is directly related to which of the following?

a. window width
b. field of view size
c. μ of H_2O
d. window level

149. Which of the following CT image archival media is capable of storing the greatest amount of information?

a. magnetic tape
b. 5¼-inch floppy disk
c. 3½-inch floppy disk
d. magnetic optical disk

150. The term ____________ describes the ability of a CT scanner to differentiate objects with minimal differences in attenuation coefficients.

a. spatial resolution
b. contrast resolution
c. linearity
d. modulation

CHAPTER 3

Simulated Exam Three

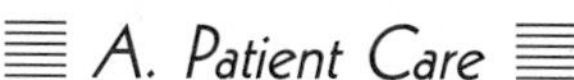

A. Patient Care

1. Which of the following symptoms indicate a vagal reaction to iodinated intravenous contrast?

1. bradycardia
2. systolic pressure of less than 80 mm Hg
3. diastolic pressure of more than 90 mm Hg

   a. 1 only
   b. 3 only
   c. 1 and 2 only
   d. 1 and 3 only

2. Before and after contact with each patient, proper hand washing requires the technologist to use soap and warm water with a circular rubbing motion for at least

   a. 10 seconds
   b. 30 seconds
   c. 2 minutes
   d. 5 minutes

3. Which of the following should be included on a patient consent form for a CT scan involving intravenous contrast media?

   a. a statement releasing the health professionals involved from any and all responsibility
   b. a clause protecting the technologist from possible lawsuit for negligence
   c. an explanation of the procedure with its accompanying risks and possible alternatives
   d. all of the above

4. The acronym PTT is used for which of the following laboratory tests?

a. prothrombin time
b. passive tachycardia test
c. partial prothrombin time
d. partial thromboplastin time

5. Which of the following is an advantage of non-ionic contrast media over ionic media?

a. decreased cost
b. decreased nephrotoxicity
c. decreased enhancement
d. decreased incidence of adverse reaction

6. Radiation exposure and its potentially harmful effects have a relationship that is termed

a. stochastic
b. nonstochastic
c. negligible
d. none of the above

7. Which of the following lists butterfly needles in decreasing order of bore dimension?

a. 19, 21, 23 gauge
b. 21, 23, 19 gauge
c. 23, 21, 19 gauge
d. 23, 19, 21 gauge

8. Which of the following is not an advantage of automatic power injectors over the manual bolus method of intravenous contrast administration?

a. uniform contrast enhancement throughout the examination
b. consistent contrast administration for all patients
c. decreased cost to the patient
d. decreased injection times

9. The maximum dose of intravenous iodinated contrast for a child should not exceed

a. 1 mg/kg body weight
b. 3 mg/kg body weight
c. 5 mg/kg body weight
d. 10 mg/kg body weight

10. The average range for normal prothrombin time is approximately

a. 3–5 seconds
b. 7–9 seconds
c. 10–12 seconds
d. 14–18 seconds

11. Examples of moderate adverse reactions to iodinated intravenous contrast media may include

1. shock
2. syncope
3. severe vomiting
   - a. 1 only
   - b. 1 and 3 only
   - c. 2 and 3 only
   - d. 1, 2, and 3

12. A typical range for skin dose to the patient during a CT study of the head is

- a. 0.1–0.3 cGy
- b. 1–2 cGy
- c. 2–4 cGy
- d. 6–8 cGy

13. The proper ratio of chest compressions to ventilations during a one-person cardiopulmonary resuscitation is

- a. 3:1
- b. 5:2
- c. 10:1
- d. 15:2

14. During intravenous drip infusion of contrast material, the contrast bottle should remain

- a. level with the patient
- b. 18–24 inches above the patient
- c. no higher than 6 inches above the patient
- d. 8–10 inches below the patient

15. Which of the following medical terms is commonly used in place of the word vomit?

- a. emesis
- b. volute
- c. fomite
- d. purulent

16. Which of the following types of isolation precautions is used to protect immunosuppressed patients from possible infection?

- a. enteric precautions
- b. strict isolation
- c. contact isolation
- d. drainage–secretion precautions

17. An intrathecal injection of iodinated contrast material may be performed for which of the following CT examinations?

- a. knee
- b. pituitary
- c. lumbar spine
- d. high-resolution chest

18. Severe reactions to intravenous iodinated contrast material occur in approximately _______________ of all patients.

a. less than 1%
b. 3%
c. 5%
d. 10%

19. The drug Solu-Cortef may be classified as which of the following?

a. anticholinergic
b. bronchodilator
c. antihistamine
d. corticosteroid

20. The injection rate of an automatic injector is set at 1.5 mL/sec. What is the injection time for a contrast volume of 150 mL?

a. 60 seconds
b. 90 seconds
c. 100 seconds
d. 120 seconds

21. Which of the following laboratory values is the most dependable measure of renal function?

a. blood urea nitrogen
b. creatinine
c. prothrombin time
d. partial thromboplastin time

22. A normal range for diastolic blood pressure in an adult is

a. 40–60 mm Hg
b. 60–90 mm Hg
c. 80–120 mm Hg
d. 95–140 mm Hg

23. While obtaining a thorough history from a patient before an intravenous injection of iodinated contrast material, which of the following topics should be included?

1. any prior allergic reactions to contrast media
2. history of infection with human immunodeficiency virus or hepatitis
3. history of asthma

a. 1 only
b. 1 and 2 only
c. 1 and 3 only
d. 1, 2, and 3

24. The escape of contrast material from a needle or blood vessel into the subcutaneous tissues is called

a. infusion
b. extraversion
c. influxation
d. extravasation

25. Patient preparation for a CT examination of the abdomen and pelvis may include which of the following?

1. receiving nothing by mouth for 4 hours before the study
2. digestion of a fatty meal 1 hour before the study
3. refraining from urination for 2 hours before the study

a. 1 only
b. 1 and 2 only
c. 2 and 3 only
d. 1, 2, and 3

26. Which of the following types of oral contrast could cause peritonitis if leakage from the digestive tract occurs due to perforation?

a. Gastrografin
b. barium sulfate
c. Hypaque
d. effervescent granules

27. Which of the following decreases patient dose during a spiral CT examination?

a. decreased scan field of view (SFOV)
b. decreased filtration
c. increased pitch
d. increased matrix size

28. A patient develops diffuse urticaria shortly after the intravenous administration of iodinated contrast media. Treatment includes

a. administration of an adrenergic drug
b. administration of intravenous fluids
c. administration of oxygen at 3–4 L/min
d. administration of an antihistamine

29. Which of the following terms is used to describe a patient having difficulty breathing?

a. dyslexia
b. dyspnea
c. dysphagia
d. dysphasia

30. The reduction in number of infectious organisms without a complete elimination is termed

a. medical asepsis
b. sterilization
c. surgical asepsis
d. immunization

B. Imaging Procedures

31. Often seen in pediatric patients, a specific type of renal mass arising from immature kidney cells is referred to as

a. Krukenberg's tumor
b. Wilms' tumor
c. von Hippel-Lindau disease
d. Ewing's sarcoma

Questions 32–34 refer to Figure 3–1.

32. Number 1 corresponds to which of the following?

a. sphenoid sinus
b. ethmoid sinus
c. frontal sinus
d. maxillary sinus

33. The section thickness that would demonstrate the greatest detail of the paranasal sinuses is

a. 3 mm
b. 5 mm
c. 7 mm
d. 10 mm

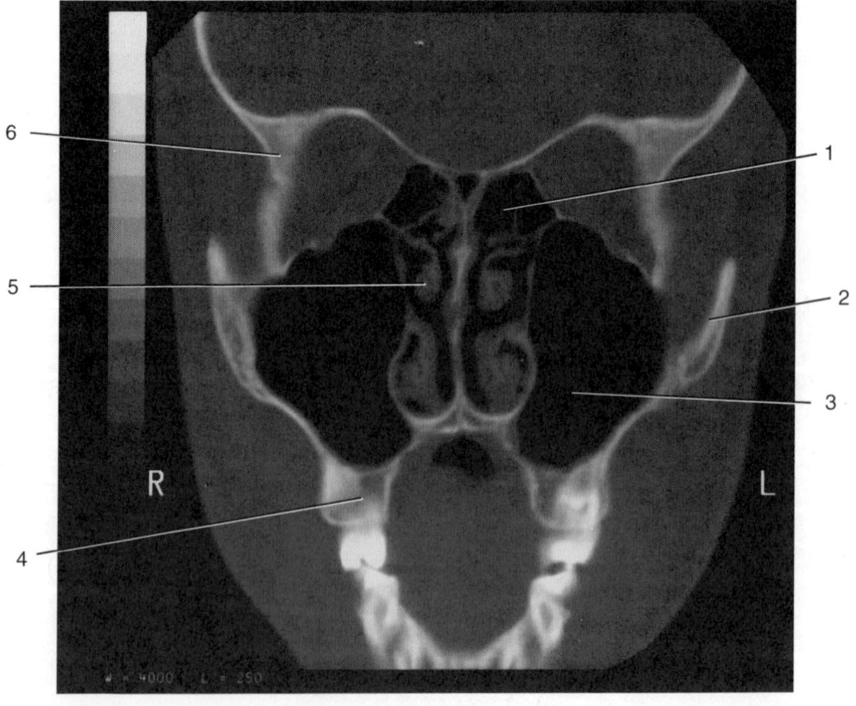

Figure 3–1.

34. Which number corresponds to the zygomatic bone?

a. 5
b. 6
c. 4
d. 2

35. During a CT examination of the abdomen using an iodinated intravenous contrast agent, which of the following abnormal findings would appear hyperdense compared with surrounding tissue?

a. angiomyolipoma of the kidney
b. hepatic cyst
c. dilated common bile duct
d. gallstone

36. Which of the following conditions would not require the injection of iodinated contrast for proper visualization during a CT examination of the brain?

a. S/P MVA 3 days previously; R/O subdural hematoma
b. headaches; R/O meningioma
c. loss of vision; R/O astrocytoma
d. lung cancer; R/O metastases

Questions 37–40 refer to Figure 3–2.

37. Number 4 corresponds to which of the following?

a. left common iliac artery
b. right common iliac artery
c. left common iliac vein
d. right common iliac vein

38. The best method for targeting the sacrum shown in the figure for closer examination is to

1. magnify the image two times
2. rescan the patient using a small SFOV
3. retrospectively reconstruct the image using a small display field of view (DFOV)

a. 1 only
b. 2 only
c. 3 only
d. 1 and 3 only

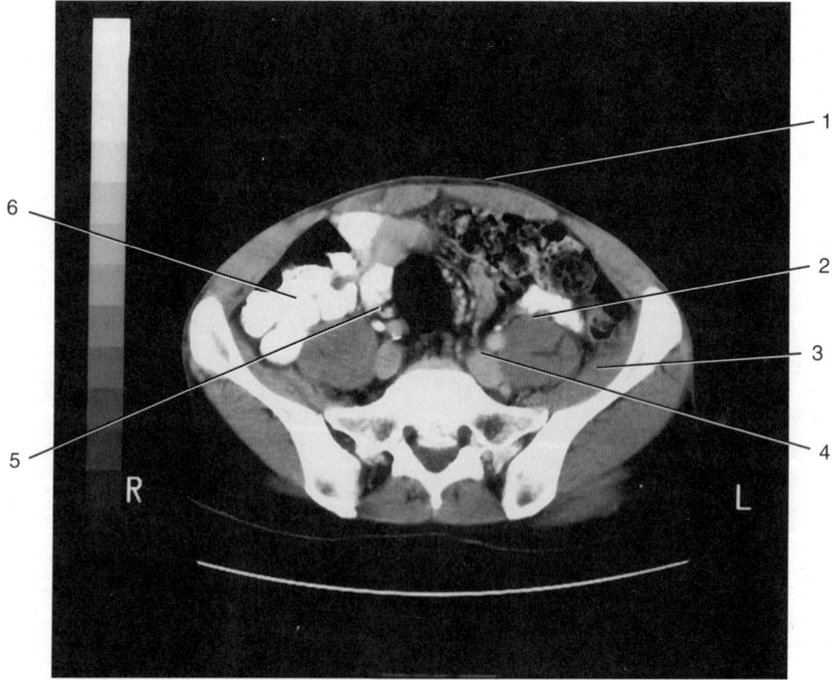

Figure 3–2.

39. Number 5 corresponds to which of the following?

a. right common iliac vein
b. right ureter
c. right common iliac artery
d. inferior mesenteric vein

40. Number 1 corresponds to which of the following?

a. psoas muscle
b. gluteus medius muscle
c. iliacus muscle
d. rectus abdominis muscle

41. Which of the following is the best scout or localizer projection for a CT scan of the neck?

a. anteroposterior
b. oblique
c. posteroanterior
d. lateral

42. Which of the following pelvic bones combine to form the acetabulum?

1. ilium
2. ischium
3. pubis

a. 2 only
b. 1 and 2 only
c. 2 and 3 only
d. 1, 2, and 3

Questions 43–46 refer to Figure 3–3.

43. Number 6 corresponds to which of the following?

a. transverse process
b. pedicle
c. lamina
d. spinous process

44. The image was formed using a large SFOV (48 cm). Which of the following DFOV sizes was used to display the image?

a. 12 cm
b. 24 cm
c. 36 cm
d. 48 cm

45. Number 2 corresponds to which of the following?

a. costotransverse articulation
b. intervertebral articulation
c. intervertebral foramen
d. costovertebral articulation

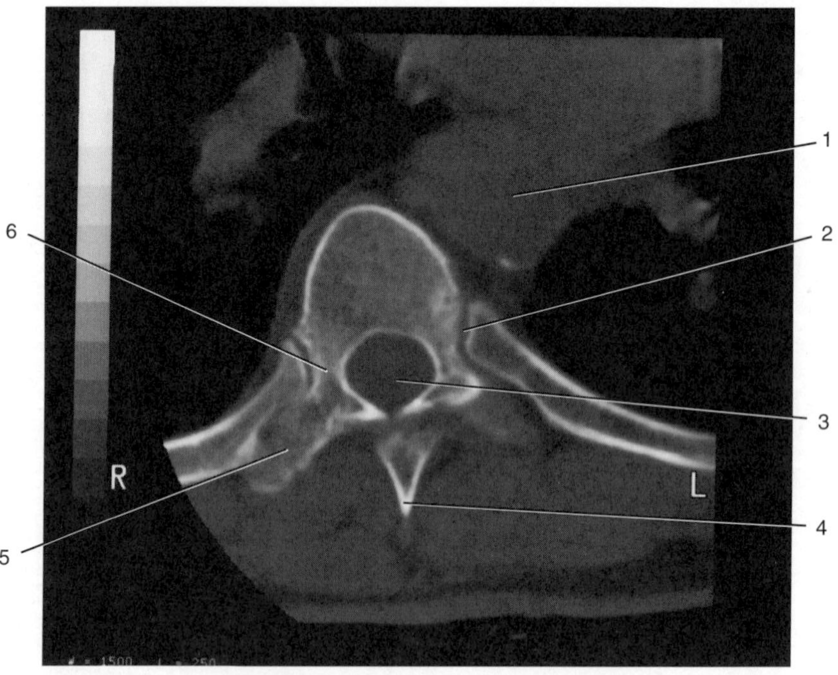

Figure 3–3.

46. Number 1 corresponds to which of the following?

a. azygos vein
b. inferior vena cava
c. descending aorta
d. esophagus

47. CT-guided needle biopsies are most commonly performed on which of the following anatomic areas?

a. breast
b. pancreas
c. cervix
d. stomach

48. Which of the following types of contrast material may be used during a CT examination of the chest?

a. diatrizoate meglumine
b. barium sulfate
c. iopamidol
d. all of the above

Questions 49–51 refer to Figure 3–4.

49. The markings labeled as number 5 correspond to which of the following?

a. atelectasis
b. interstitial pulmonary disease
c. pulmonary hilum
d. emphysema

50. The presence of the board or flat tabletop as shown by number 4 indicates that this is what type of CT study?

a. quantitative
b. radiation planning
c. invasive
d. general survey

51. Number 2 most likely corresponds to which of the following?

a. asbestosis
b. tumor
c. pleural effusion
d. sarcoidosis

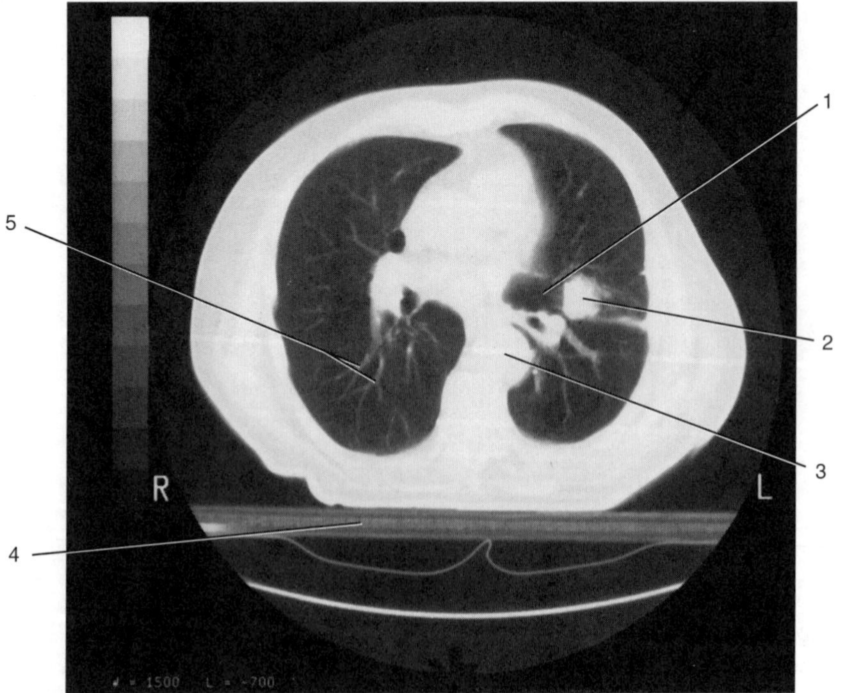

Figure 3–4.

52. Which of the following statements regarding the pituitary gland is false?

a. It is sometimes referred to as the hypophysis cerebri.
b. It is seated within the sella turcica.
c. The infundibulum attaches it to the hypothalamus.
d. It is responsible for the production of epinephrine.

53. Which of the following sets of section widths and spacing would be best suited for a general survey CT study of the abdomen and pelvis on a patient with a history of lymphoma?

a. 3 × 3 mm
b. 5 × 15 mm
c. 10 × 15 mm
d. 10 × 30 mm

Questions 54–57 refer to Figure 3–5.

54. Which number corresponds to the trapezius muscle?

a. 4
b. 3
c. 6
d. none of the above

55. An adequate volume of intravenous contrast for this CT examination of the neck would be

a. 25 mL
b. 50 mL
c. 125 mL
d. 225 mL

56. Number 1 corresponds to which of the following?

a. common carotid artery
b. external jugular vein
c. internal jugular vein
d. brachiocephalic artery

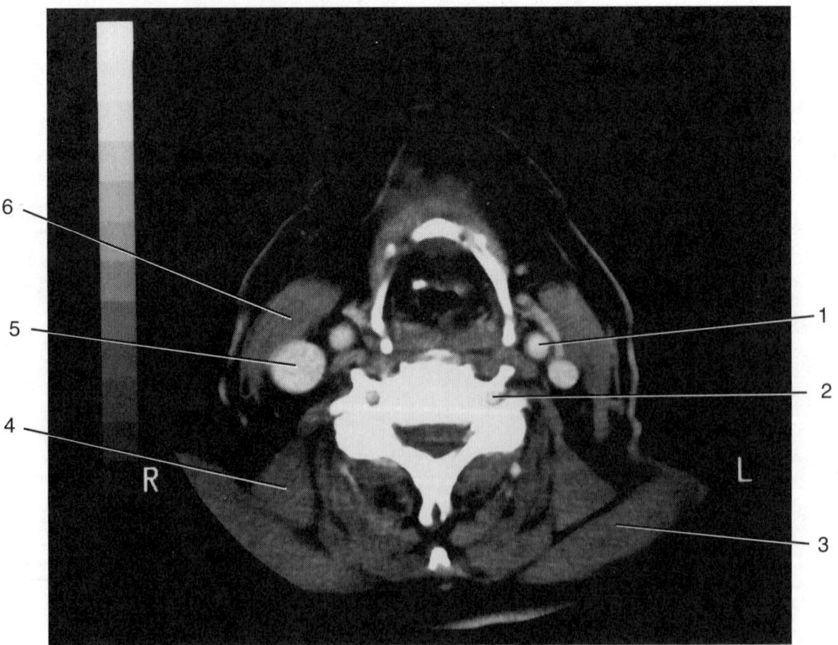

Figure 3–5.

57. Number 4 corresponds to which of the following?

a. erector spinae muscle
b. rhomboid major muscle
c. deltoid muscle
d. levator scapulae muscle

58. The kidneys are located in the retroperitoneum and are bound by a band of fibrous connective tissue called

a. Cooper's ligament
b. fascia of Camper
c. linea alba
d. Gerota's fascia

59. Which of the following terms is used to describe a rapidly obtained CT scan with minimized interscan delays?

a. ultrafast
b. dynamic
c. standard
d. static

Questions 60–62 refer to Figure 3–6.

60. The imaging plane used to form the image of the foot was which of the following?
   a. coronal
   b. axial
   c. sagittal
   d. oblique

61. Number 1 corresponds to which of the following?
   a. first metatarsal
   b. second metatarsal
   c. third metatarsal
   d. fourth metatarsal

62. Number 2 corresponds to which of the following?
   a. proximal phalanges
   b. lateral and medial cuneiforms
   c. sesamoid bones
   d. bone spurs

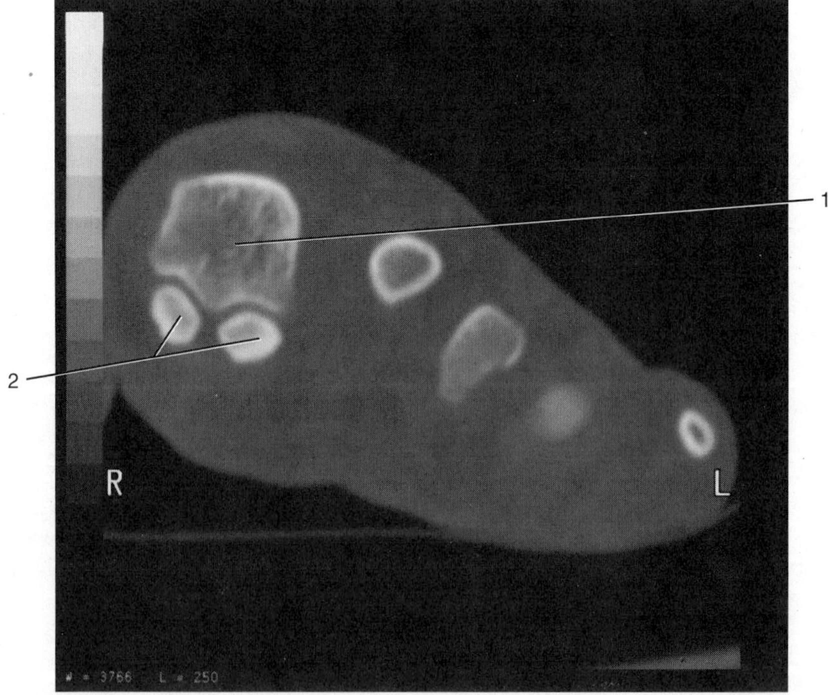

Figure 3–6.

63. The water-soluble oral contrast agents used for CT scans of the abdomen and pelvis should contain approximately _______________ iodine.

a. 2%–5%
b. 8%–12%
c. 15%–20%
d. 25%–40%

Questions 64–66 refer to Figure 3–7.

64. Which number corresponds to the superior mesenteric vein?

a. 3
b. 5
c. 1
d. 2

65. Number 4 corresponds to which of the following?

a. descending colon
b. spleen
c. adrenal gland
d. renal vein

66. Number 6 corresponds to which of the following?

a. duodenum
b. terminal ileum
c. appendix
d. pancreas

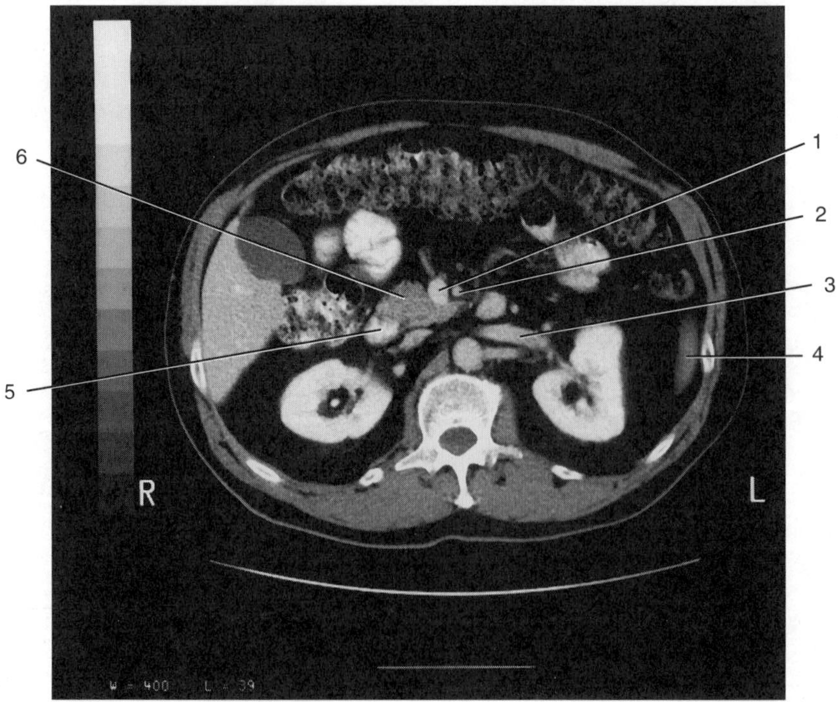

Figure 3–7.

67. Which of the following correctly describes the patient position relative to the gantry for a CT study of the brain?

a. supine, feet first
b. prone, feet first
c. supine, head first
d. prone, head first

68. A CT examination of the lumbar spine reveals a herniated disk at the level of L2–L3. Which of the following reformat planes would best demonstrate the posterior compression of the disk material onto the spinal cord?

a. coronal
b. sagittal
c. axial
d. oblique

69. Which of the following algorithm types provides the greatest soft-tissue detail during a CT study of the pelvis?

a. high spatial frequency
b. detail
c. edge
d. low spatial frequency

70. Which of the following pathologic processes is an interstitial disease of the lungs?

a. bronchiectasis
b. mediastinal lymphadenopathy
c. pulmonary metastasis
d. bronchogenic carcinoma

Questions 71–74 refer to Figure 3–8.

71. What procedure is being performed in the figure?
- a. quantitative CT
- b. percutaneous abscess drainage
- c. percutaneous needle biopsy
- d. radiation therapy planning

72. Number 4 corresponds to which of the following?
- a. streaking artifact
- b. hernia
- c. gunshot wound
- d. biopsy needle

73. Number 3 corresponds to which of the following?
- a. abscess
- b. hepatic tumor
- c. ascending colon
- d. gallbladder

74. Number 1 corresponds to which of the following?
- a. transverse colon
- b. splenic flexure
- c. stomach
- d. diverticular abscess

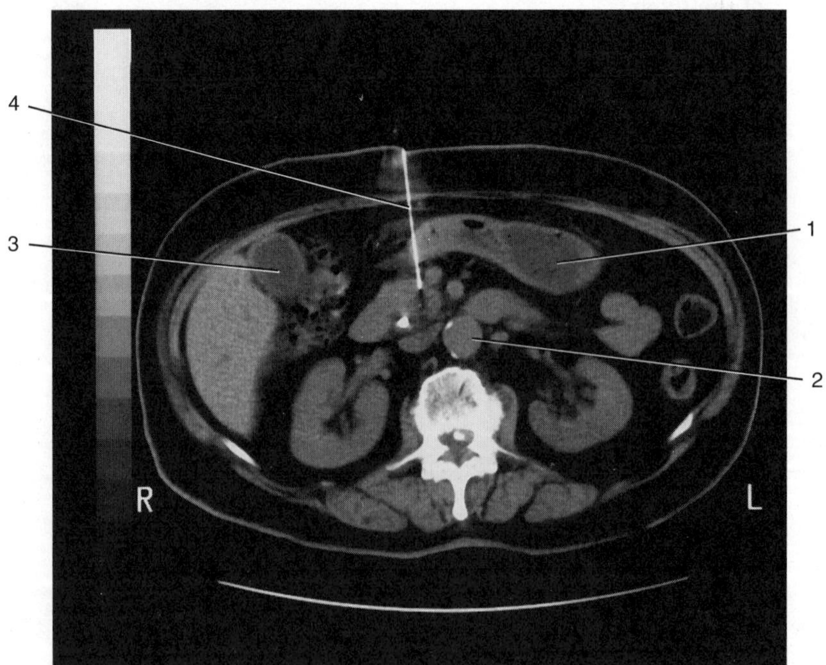

Figure 3–8.

75. Cerebrospinal fluid is produced in the

a. tentorium cerebelli
b. pineal gland
c. corpus callosum
d. choroid plexuses

76. The accumulation of gas within a degenerating intervertebral disk is called the

a. aeration effect
b. vacuum phenomenon
c. oxygen saturation point
d. carbonization sign

Questions 77–80 refer to Figure 3–9.

77. Which of the following are accurate methods of centering this patient's hip within the gantry?

1. Palpate approximately 6 inches below the iliac crest.
2. Have the patient rotate the leg and palpate the greater trochanter.
3. Palpate the pubic bone.

a. 1 and 2 only
b. 1 and 3 only
c. 2 and 3 only
d. 1, 2, and 3

78. Number 3 corresponds to which of the following?

a. pubis
b. ilium
c. ischium
d. lesser trochanter

79. Which number corresponds to the acetabulum?

a. 5
b. 3
c. 1
d. 2

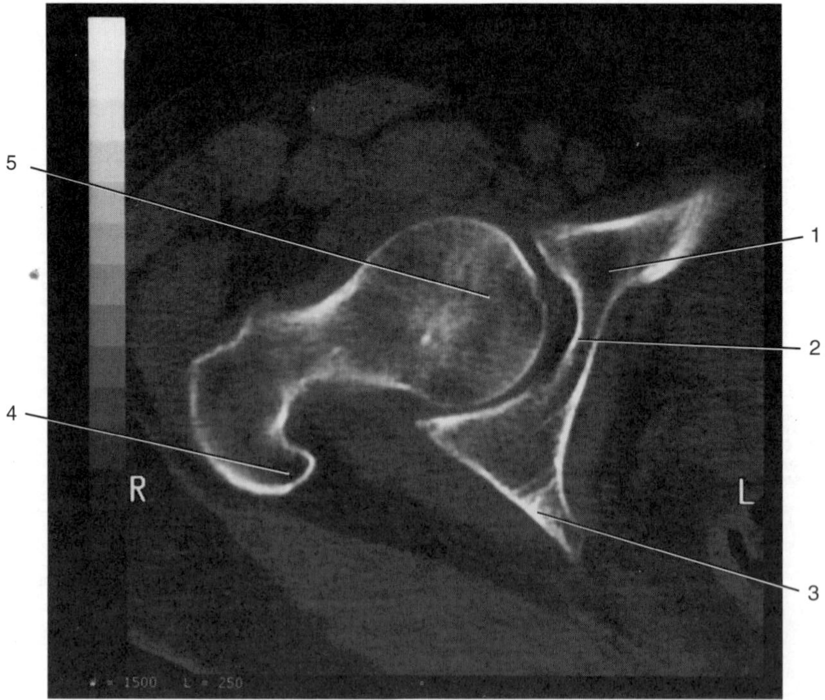

Figure 3–9.

80. Number 1 corresponds to which of the following?

a. pubis
b. ischium
c. tuberosity of ischium
d. ilium

81. A stereotactic unit is used for which of the following specialized CT examinations?

a. CT-guided fine-needle aspiration of an abdominal abscess
b. three-dimensional CT angiogram
c. CT-guided biopsy of the brain
d. dual window scanning

82. Accurate demonstration of ______________ would most likely require the intravenous injection of iodinated contrast during a CT study of the chest.

a. pneumonia
b. sarcoidosis
c. a dissecting aortic aneurysm
d. a solitary pulmonary nodule

Questions 83–86 refer to Figure 3–10.

83. Number 2 corresponds to which of the following?
   a. azygos vein
   b. esophagus
   c. internal jugular vein
   d. descending aorta

84. Number 4 corresponds to which of the following?
   a. first rib
   b. second rib
   c. clavicle
   d. acromion

85. Number 1 corresponds to which of the following?
   a. thyroid cartilage
   b. hyoid bone
   c. Adam's apple
   d. thyroid gland

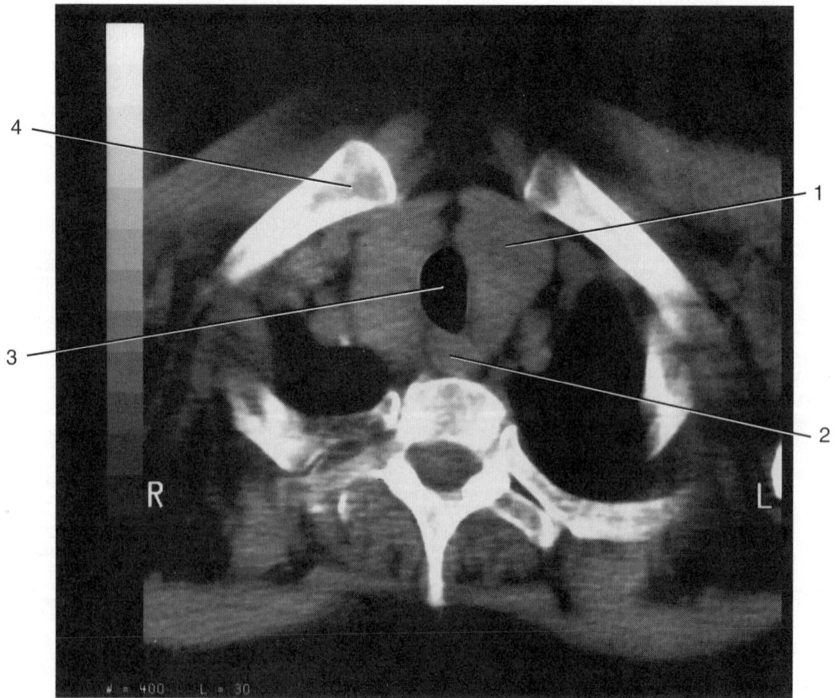

Figure 3–10.

86. Which of the following pathologic processes best describes the abnormal finding shown in the figure?

a. primary lung cancer
b. esophageal tumor
c. enlarged thyroid
d. tonsillitis

87. A double-contrast CT study of the bladder in a female patient includes an intravenous injection of iodinated contrast and

a. 300 mL of diatrizoate sodium administered via the rectum
b. 750–1000 mL of diatrizoate meglumine administered orally the evening before the study
c. the insertion of a tampon into the vagina
d. 100 mL of diluted diatrizoate meglumine and 100 mL of air administered into the bladder via a Foley catheter

88. Demonstration of a thoracic intervertebral disk of a patient with severe lateral scoliosis may be improved by

a. increasing the mAs used
b. placing the patient in the prone position
c. angling the gantry inferiorly or superiorly
d. placing the patient in a lateral decubitus position and angling the gantry

Questions 89–93 refer to Figure 3–11.

89. Number 2 corresponds to which of the following?
  a. erector spinae muscle
  b. gluteus medius muscle
  c. psoas major muscle
  d. sacrospinalis muscle

90. The circle labeled as number 1 is used here for what purpose?
  a. to outline an area of pathology
  b. to make a region of interest measurement
  c. to target an area for needle biopsy
  d. to change the DFOV

91. The measured density of the area labeled as number 4 is approximately +5 Hounsfield units. This most likely represents
  a. a kidney stone
  b. an angiomyolipoma
  c. a renal tumor
  d. a renal cyst

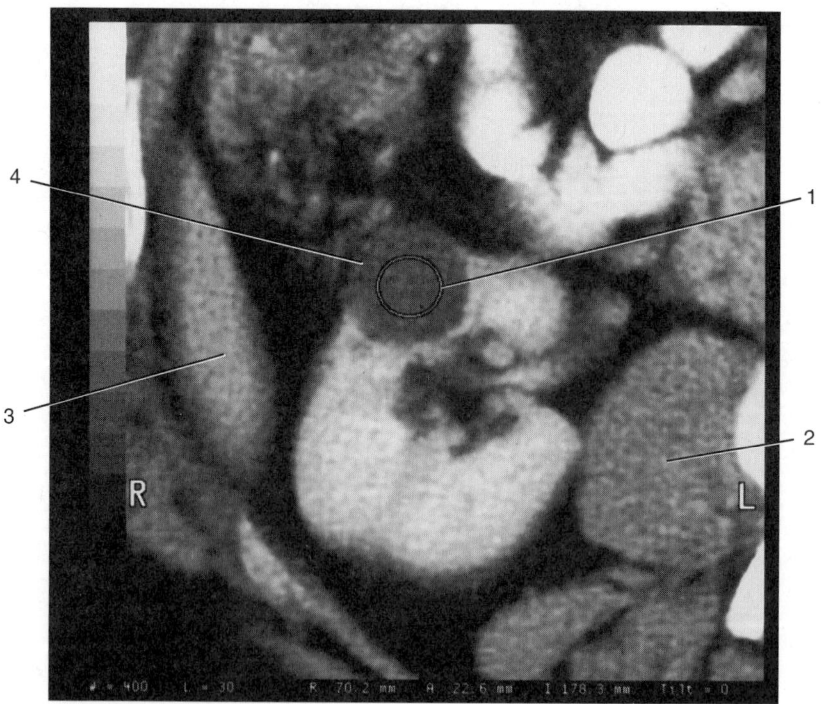

Figure 3–11.

92. Which of the following statements is true concerning CT scans of the abdomen for the differentiation of renal cysts?

1. Scans should be done through the kidneys before and after intravenous contrast administration.
2. Region of interest measurements of the cyst should be made to help determine its composition.
3. The patient should refrain from urination for 2 hours before the examination.

a. 1 only
b. 1 and 2 only
c. 2 and 3 only
d. 1, 2, and 3

93. Number 3 corresponds to which of the following?

a. adrenal gland
b. spleen
c. liver
d. duodenum

94. Which of the following correctly describes the position of the seminal vesicles in the male pelvis?

a. posterior to the bladder and anterior to the rectum
b. superior to the rectum and inferior to the prostate
c. anterior to the bladder and superior to the prostate
d. inferior to the bladder and posterior to the rectum

Questions 95–98 refer to Figure 3–12.

95. The localizer (scout) image was performed for a general CT survey of the chest. What technical errors were made with this image?

1. Image proceeds too far superiorly and inferiorly.
2. Incorrect azimuth is used.
3. Patient's hands should be positioned overhead.

a. 1 only
b. 1 and 2 only
c. 1 and 3 only
d. 1, 2, and 3

96. Number 1 corresponds to which of the following?

a. acromion
b. coronoid
c. coracoid
d. olecranon

97. Number 4 corresponds to which of the following?

a. esophagus
b. middle hemidiaphragm
c. carina
d. thymus gland

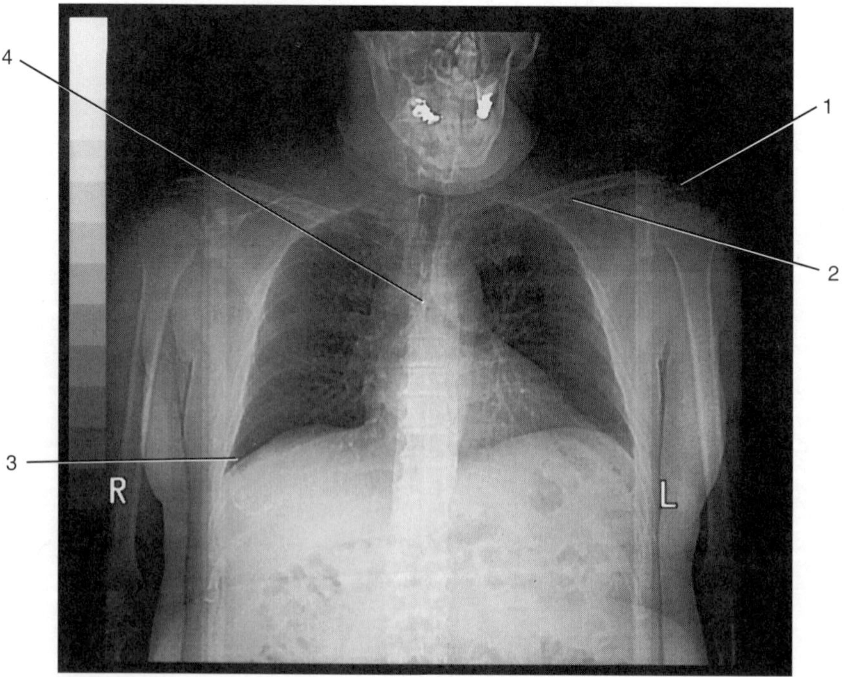

Figure 3–12.

98. Number 3 corresponds to which of the following?

a. cardiophrenic angle
b. costophrenic angle
c. caudal margin of pleura
d. lingula

99. The prone position may be used for a post-myelogram CT examination of the lumbar spine in an effort to

a. reduce the lordotic curve
b. decrease patient gonadal dose
c. reduce metrizamide pooling
d. increase the lordotic curve

100. During a CT examination of a female pelvis for a suspected malignancy, ascites may be present in an area posterior to the uterus and ovaries known as

a. the cul-de-sac
b. Morison's pouch
c. the space of Retzius
d. the prevesicle compartment

Questions 101–105 refer to Figure 3–13.

101. Which number corresponds to the lateral rectus muscle?
   a. 5
   b. 2
   c. 6
   d. none of the above

102. Number 4 corresponds to which of the following?
   a. frontal sinus
   b. maxillary sinus
   c. sphenoid sinus
   d. ethmoid sinus

103. The image is part of a series that could be used to evaluate which of the following?
1. posterior fossa
2. orbits
3. paranasal sinuses
   a. 1 only
   b. 1 and 3 only
   c. 2 and 3 only
   d. 1, 2, and 3

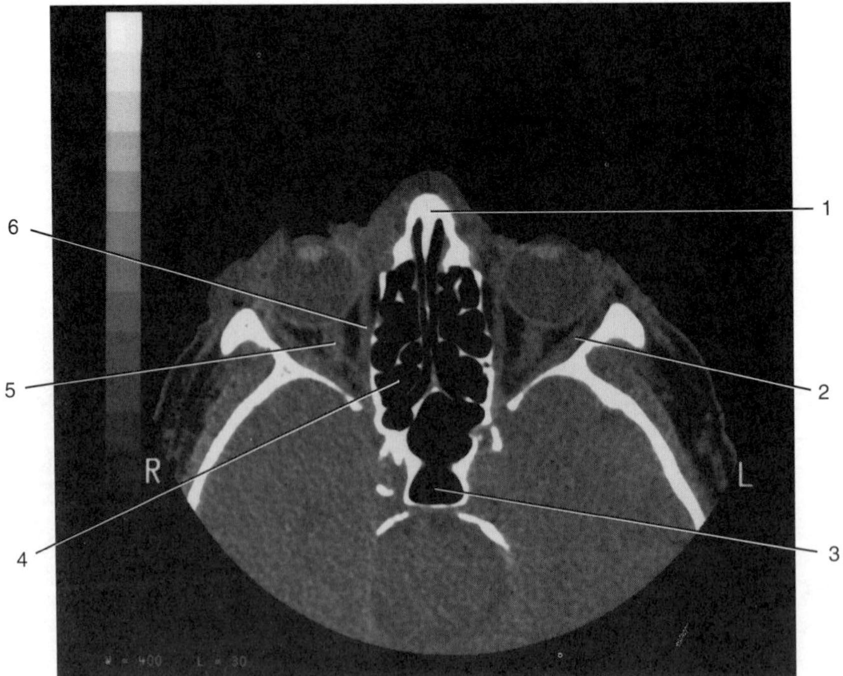

Figure 3–13.

104. Number 5 corresponds to which of the following?

a. superior rectus muscle
b. levator palpebrae superioris muscle
c. optic nerve
d. inferior rectus muscle

105. Number 1 corresponds to which of the following?

a. vomer
b. nasal bone
c. lacrimal bone
d. clivus

C. Physics and Instrumentation

106. First-generation CT scanners possess which of the following characteristics?

a. pencil-thin x-ray beam
b. silver halide detectors
c. rotate–rotate geometry
d. nutating detector array

107. The average CT value for blood is approximately

a. −50 Hounsfield units
b. 0 Hounsfield units
c. +45 Hounsfield units
d. +100 Hounsfield units

108. Before a CT image can be reconstructed by a computer, the transmission signal produced by the detectors must be converted into numeric information by a(n)

a. kernel
b. analog-to-digital converter
c. array processor
d. digital-to-analog converter

109. The dimensions of a voxel may be calculated as the product of which of the following?

a. matrix size and pixel size
b. pixel size and section width
c. DFOV and matrix size
d. DFOV and pixel size

110. A voxel whose attenuation coefficient is less than that of water is assigned a pixel value with a(n) ______________ CT number.

a. positive
b. extremely large
c. negative
d. none of the above

111. Which of the following terms are commonly used to describe the ability of a CT scanner to differentiate objects with similar linear attenuation coefficients?

1. spatial resolution
2. sensitivity
3. contrast resolution

a. 1 only
b. 3 only
c. 1 and 2 only
d. 2 and 3 only

112. Which of the following section widths would cause the greatest amount of partial volume averaging?

a. 1 mm
b. 3 mm
c. 5 mm
d. 10 mm

113. Which of the following factors has no measurable effect on spatial resolution?

a. focal spot size
b. kVp
c. detector sampling frequency
d. matrix size

114. An image that is reconstructed a second time with some change in technical factor is termed _______________ .

a. reiterated
b. post-processed
c. retrospective
d. reformatted

115. Cupping artifacts most commonly occur in the

a. chest
b. abdomen
c. pelvis
d. brain

116. What matrix size is used to reconstruct an image with a DFOV of 25 cm and a pixel area of 0.25 mm^2?

a. 80 × 80 pixels
b. 256 × 256 pixels
c. 320 × 320 pixels
d. 512 × 512 pixels

117. The assignment of different generations to CT scanners is based on the configuration of the

a. patient and gantry
b. tube and detectors
c. anode and cathode
d. tube and collimators

118. Which of the following types of image noise can be most easily reduced by the CT technologist?

a. electronic noise
b. artifactual noise
c. quantum noise
d. detector noise

119. Which of the following types of image reconstruction was used in the first-generation prototype CT scanner?

a. convolution method
b. iterative technique
c. Fourier transform
d. back-projection

120. A CT image is displayed in a window with a level of 0 and a width of 500. Which of the following statements is correct?

a. Pixels with values between 0 and 500 Hounsfield units appear white.
b. Pixels with values between −250 and +250 Hounsfield units are assigned shades of gray.
c. Pixels with values greater than +500 Hounsfield units are black.
d. Pixels with negative values appear white.

121. During CT angiography, images may be reconstructed using only the greatest density encountered along each ray. This type of specialized CT image is called a(n)

a. three-dimensional model
b. volume-rendered image
c. MIP image
d. surface-rendered image

122. The ability of a CT scanner to image a small high-density object is controlled by the ________________ of the scanner.

a. contrast resolution
b. spatial resolution
c. sensitivity
d. contrast resolution and sensitivity

123. Which of the following artifacts is not affected by the CT technologist?
a. motion
b. partial volume
c. edge gradient
d. ring

124. Which of the following quality control tests should be frequently performed on a CT scanner?
1. The CT number calibration should be checked.
2. The noise levels (standard deviation) of a water phantom should be examined.
3. The accuracy of the laser-localization device should be tested.

a. 1 only
b. 1 and 2 only
c. 1 and 3 only
d. 1, 2, and 3

125. The average photon energy of the CT x-ray beam can be increased by
a. increasing mAs
b. increasing filtration
c. increasing collimation
d. all of the above

Questions 126–128 refer to Figure 3–14.

126. The streaking artifact shown in the figure is most likely due to
a. detector malfunction
b. tube arcing
c. beam hardening
d. out-of-field errors

127. Which of the following types of algorithms is best suited to demonstrate the bony details of this shoulder joint?
a. high spatial frequency
b. soft tissue
c. standard
d. low spatial frequency

128. Which of the following window levels was most likely used to display the image?
a. −700 Hounsfield units
b. 0 Hounsfield units
c. +50 Hounsfield units
d. +250 Hounsfield units

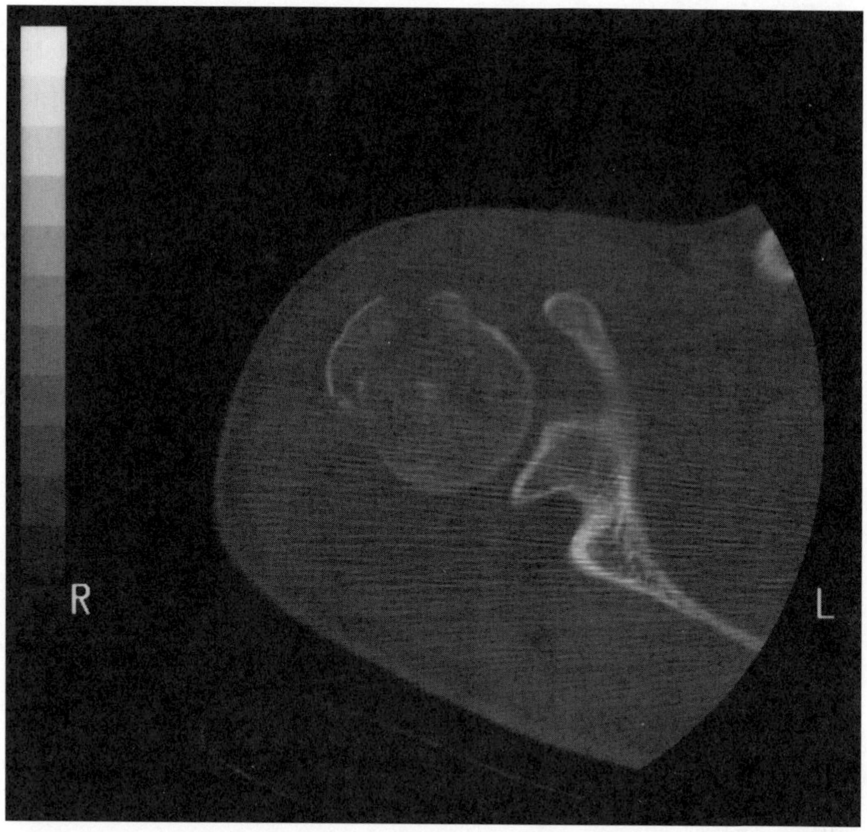

Figure 3–14.

129. The largest disruptor of the contrast resolution of a CT scanner is
   a. patient motion
   b. noise
   c. hardware malfunction
   d. beam hardening

130. CT images that have been reconstructed from a portion of the data acquisition process in the hopes of reducing patient motion artifacts are called
   a. dynamic images
   b. subtraction images
   c. segmented images
   d. filtered images

131. When using a third-generation CT scanner, it is important that reference detectors positioned at the peripheral portions of the detector array be exposed to

a. homogeneous radiation
b. unattenuated radiation
c. monochromatic radiation
d. remnant radiation

132. Which of the following is capable of causing an edge gradient artifact?

a. detector malfunction
b. involuntary patient motion
c. dense bone
d. tube arcing

133. Third-generation CT scanners use which of the following scan geometric relationships?

a. translate–rotate
b. rotate–stationary
c. translate–axial
d. rotate–rotate

134. The spatial resolution of a CT scanner is often measured using the MTF, which is an acronym for

a. maximum transmissivity frequency
b. modulation target function
c. minimum transmissivity frequency
d. modulation transfer function

Questions 135–137 refer to Figure 3–15.

135. Which of the following terms best describes the artifact shown?
   a. edge gradient
   b. Gibbs phenomenon
   c. density gradient
   d. partial volume

136. The artifact is most likely caused by
   a. involuntary motion
   b. aliasing
   c. surgical staples
   d. tube arcing

137. The patient scanned measured 38 cm across. An appropriate DFOV for the display of this image is
   a. 30 cm
   b. 40 cm
   c. 44 cm
   d. 48 cm

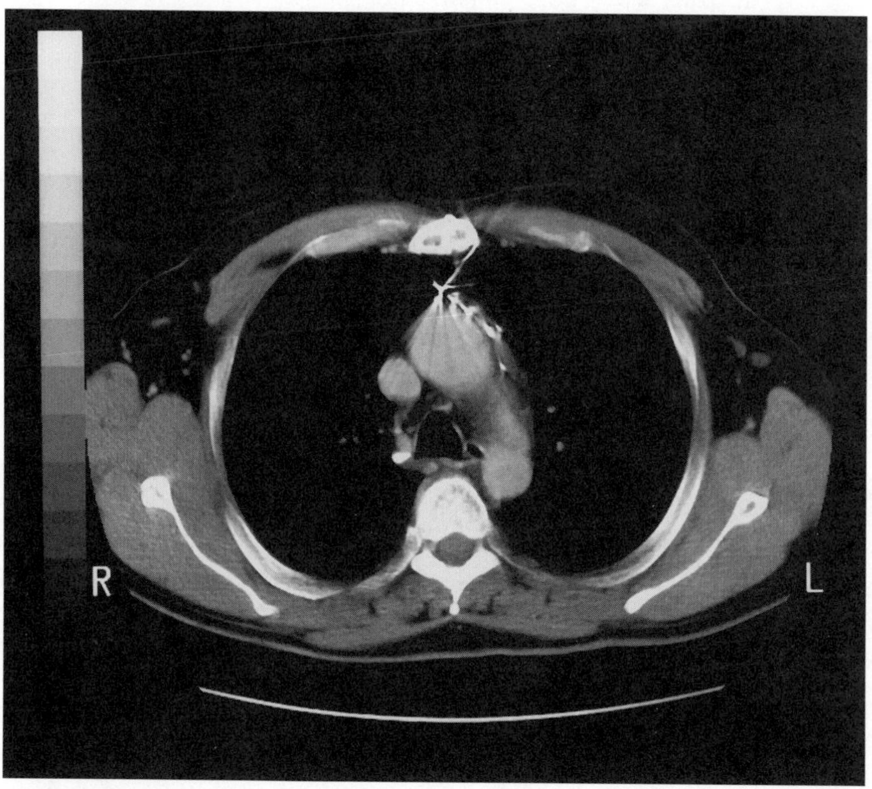

Figure 3–15.

138. In 1979, the scientists ______________ shared the Nobel Prize for their research in CT.

a. Watson and Crick
b. Olendorf and Hounsfield
c. Hounsfield and Cormack
d. Hounsfield and Ambrose

139. Areas of a CT image containing abrupt changes in tissue density are electronically represented by

a. positive CT numbers
b. high spatial frequencies
c. negative CT numbers
d. low spatial frequencies

140. Which of the following formulas may be used to calculate the dimensions of a pixel?

a. pixel size = matrix size/DFOV
b. pixel size = DFOV × matrix size
c. pixel size = slice thickness/matrix
d. pixel size = DFOV/matrix size

141. The smallest unit of information used in the binary language of computers is the

a. bit
b. chip
c. base
d. byte

142. A CT scanner measures the linear attenuation coefficient of a voxel of tissue to be 0.40. The linear attenuation coefficient of water for this scanner equals 0.20. The CT number assigned to the pixel representing this voxel of tissue equals

a. −1000 Hounsfield units
b. 0 Hounsfield units
c. 1 Hounsfield unit
d. +1000 Hounsfield units

143. The intensity of the x-ray beam after it passes through an object to a detector is called the

a. incident intensity
b. ray
c. transmitted intensity
d. primary beam

144. Which of the following statements regarding predetector collimation of the CT x-ray beam is true?

a. Predetector collimation reduces patient dose.
b. Predetector collimation reduces the production of scatter radiation.
c. Predetector collimation controls the section thickness of a CT scan.
d. Predetector collimation removes scatter radiation before it reaches the detectors.

Questions 145–147 refer to Figure 3–16.

145. The streaking artifacts were most likely caused by

a. tube arcing
b. dental fillings
c. detector malfunction
d. insufficient technique

146. Which of the following steps would reduce the artifact?

1. reduce the section thickness
2. angle the gantry around fillings
3. decrease kVp

a. 1 only
b. 2 only
c. 3 only
d. 2 and 3 only

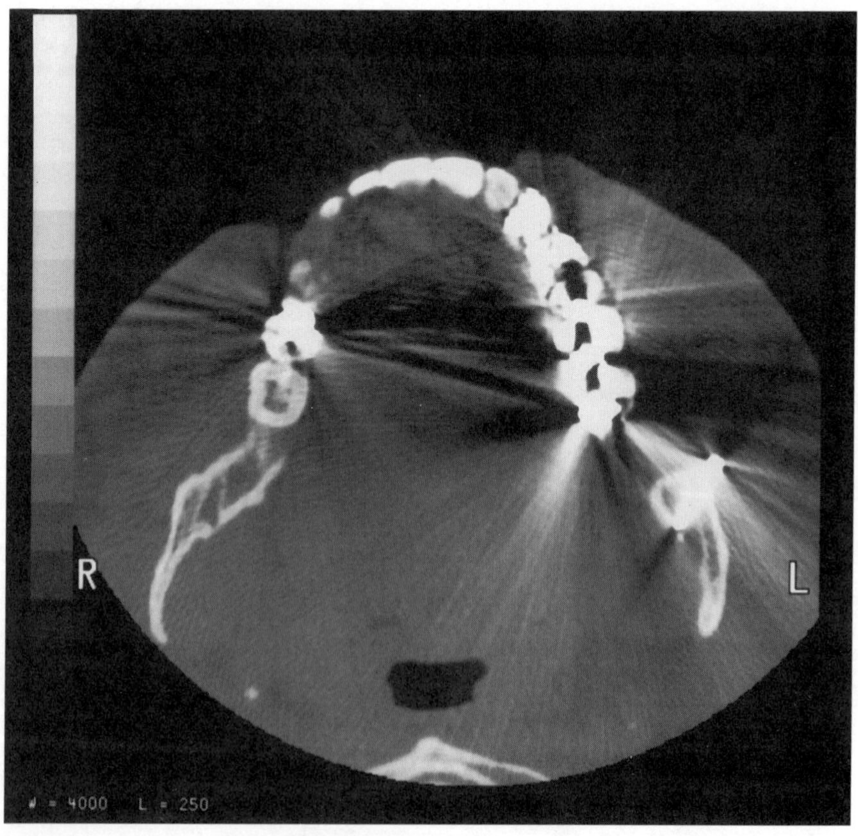

Figure 3–16.

147. The image was produced with a 1.0-mm aperture size and was displayed using a 512^2 matrix and a 15-cm DFOV. The voxel dimension for this image is

a. 0.29 mm × 0.29 mm × 1.0 mm
b. 2.9 mm × 2.9 mm × 1.0 mm
c. 3.4 mm × 3.4 mm × 1.0 mm
d. 0.29 mm × 0.29 mm × 1.0 cm

148. Which of the following technical adjustments would decrease the quantum noise of a CT image?

1. increased mAs
2. decreased section width
3. increased section width

a. 1 only
b. 1 and 2 only
c. 1 and 3 only
d. none of the above

149. Which of the following would magnify the CT image on the display monitor?

a. decreased matrix size
b. increased SFOV
c. decreased DFOV
d. increased DFOV

150. A CT scanner with a limiting resolution of 15 lp/cm can resolve an object as small as

a. 0.1 mm
b. 0.3 mm
c. 0.6 mm
d. 1.0 mm

CHAPTER 4

Simulated Exam Four

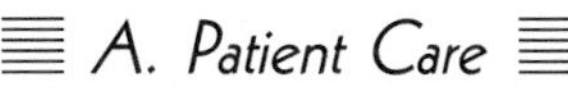

A. Patient Care

1. The normal pulse rate range in a child is

a. 30–50 beats per minute
b. 60–100 beats per minute
c. 70–120 beats per minute
d. 110–150 beats per minute

2. Which of the following are signs or symptoms of hypovolemic shock?

1. hypertension
2. oliguria
3. pallor

a. 1 only
b. 1 and 3 only
c. 2 and 3 only
d. 1, 2, and 3

3. Which of the following would not be used as a site for the injection of iodinated contrast material?

a. cephalic vein
b. brachial artery
c. antecubital vein
d. basilic vein

4. Which of the following technical changes would decrease patient dose during a CT examination?

a. decreased matrix size
b. change from soft tissue to bone algorithm
c. decreased tube rotation from 360° to 180°
d. decreased display field of view (DFOV)

5. Parenteral routes of medication administration include which of the following?
1. subcutaneous
2. intradermal
3. transdermal
   a. 1 only
   b. 1 and 2 only
   c. 2 and 3 only
   d. 1, 2, and 3

6. The viscosity of a contrast material may be decreased through
   a. increases in pressure
   b. decreases in temperature
   c. decreases in volume
   d. increases in temperature

7. Which of the following is an example of a mild reaction to iodinated intravenous contrast media?
   a. dyspnea
   b. shock
   c. pulmonary edema
   d. vomiting

8. The patient is not required to give informed consent for which of the following CT studies?
   a. noncontrast brain study to rule out subdural hematoma
   b. CT-guided abscess drainage
   c. stereotactic biopsy of a cranial tumor
   d. MPR imaging of the shoulder

9. Which of the following is a non-ionic contrast material?
   a. iodamide
   b. iothalamate
   c. iohexol
   d. diatrizoate

10. A patient's blood pressure is measured as 140/70 mm Hg. The number 140 represents
   a. the pressure within the arterial vessels during contraction of the heart
   b. the pressure exerted on the chambers of the heart while the heart is relaxed
   c. the pressure within the arterial vessels while the heart is relaxed
   d. the pressure exerted on the chambers of the heart during contraction of the heart

11. Which of the following medications may be administered to a patient having a severe anaphylactoid reaction to iodinated contrast material?

1. epinephrine
2. atropine
3. diphenhydramine
   - a. 1 only
   - b. 1 and 2 only
   - c. 1 and 3 only
   - d. 1, 2, and 3

12. A non-ionic intravenous contrast agent has an average osmolality of

- a. 300 mOsm/kg water
- b. 750 mOsm/kg water
- c. 1300 mOsm/kg water
- d. 3000 mOsm/kg water

13. The addition of ______________ makes an autoclave more efficient at sterilization than an oven.

- a. antiseptic solution
- b. moisture
- c. extreme pressure
- d. ultraviolet light

14. An average range for activated partial thromboplastin time is

- a. 10–12 seconds
- b. 17–21 seconds
- c. 28–34 seconds
- d. 43–55 seconds

15. In a female patient, gonadal shielding may be applied during which of the following CT examinations?

1. chest
2. abdomen
3. brain
   - a. 3 only
   - b. 1 and 2 only
   - c. 2 and 3 only
   - d. 1, 2, and 3

16. The first step in providing cardiopulmonary resuscitation is always

- a. to give 15 chest compressions
- b. to clear the airway
- c. to call for help
- d. to begin rescue breathing

17. A suction unit used on a patient with a chest tube should always remain

- a. below the patient
- b. level with the patient
- c. above the patient
- d. none of the above

18. A total volume of 125 mL of iodinated intravenous contrast is administered via automatic injector in 50 seconds. The flow rate for this injection is

a. 0.75 mL/sec
b. 1.25 mL/sec
c. 1.75 mL/sec
d. 2.5 mL/sec

19. Which of the following devices is used to measure the patient dose from a CT examination?

a. Geiger-Müller counter
b. thermoluminescent dosimeter
c. ionization chamber
d. film badge

20. Which of the following is not an absolute contraindication of intravenous contrast administration?

a. sickle cell anemia in active crisis
b. elevated serum creatinine level
c. pheochromocytoma
d. allergic history to shellfish

21. Patient preparation for a contrast-enhanced CT examination of the chest should include

a. nothing by mouth for 4 hours before the examination
b. low-residue diet for 12–24 hours before the examination
c. cleansing enema on the day preceding the examination
d. no preparation

22. The quantity of radiation dose received by the patient from a series of CT scans is referred to as the

a. MSAD
b. XCAL
c. CTDI
d. MTF

23. Which of the following iodinated contrasts may be used for an intrathecal injection?

a. meglumine
b. iodipamide
c. iohexol
d. sodium-meglumine diatrizoate

24. Which of the following sizes of butterfly needles allows for the most rapid administration of iodinated intravenous contrast media?

a. 19 gauge
b. 21 gauge
c. 23 gauge
d. 25 gauge

25. A patient is scheduled for a intravenous iodinated contrast-enhanced CT scan of the kidneys. Before the injection, the involved medical personnel should examine recently measured laboratory values for which of the following?

1. complete blood count
2. creatinine
3. prothrombin time
   a. 2 only
   b. 3 only
   c. 1 and 2 only
   d. 2 and 3 only

26. Which of the following terms may be used to indicate a feeling of faintness?

   a. lethargy
   b. synergy
   c. anosmia
   d. syncope

27. Which of the following types of isolation techniques protects against infection transmitted through fecal material?

   a. acid-fast bacillus isolation
   b. contact isolation
   c. enteric precautions
   d. drainage-secretion precautions

28. Which of the following laboratory values is used to measure the coagulation ability of a patient before an invasive CT study?

1. partial thromboplastin time
2. hematocrit
3. prothrombin time
   a. 1 only
   b. 1 and 3 only
   c. 2 and 3 only
   d. 1, 2, and 3

29. Which of the following types of central venous lines may be used for the administration of iodinated contrast with an automatic injector?

   a. Infuse-A-Port
   b. Hickman catheter
   c. port-A-Cath
   d. none of the above

30. Which of the following intravenous contrast administration methods provides the greatest overall plasma–iodine concentration?

   a. drip infusion
   b. bolus technique
   c. biphasic technique
   d. CT portography

B. Imaging Procedures

31. High-resolution CT is most commonly used for the evaluation of the

a. pancreas
b. brain
c. lungs
d. mediastinum

32. During a CT-guided needle biopsy, the needle insertion site is usually anesthetized with

a. diazepam
b. lidocaine
c. lithium
d. oxycodone HCl (Percodan)

Questions 33–37 refer to Figure 4–1.

33. Number 4 corresponds to which of the following?

a. greater trochanter
b. sciatic tubercle
c. lesser trochanter
d. coracoid

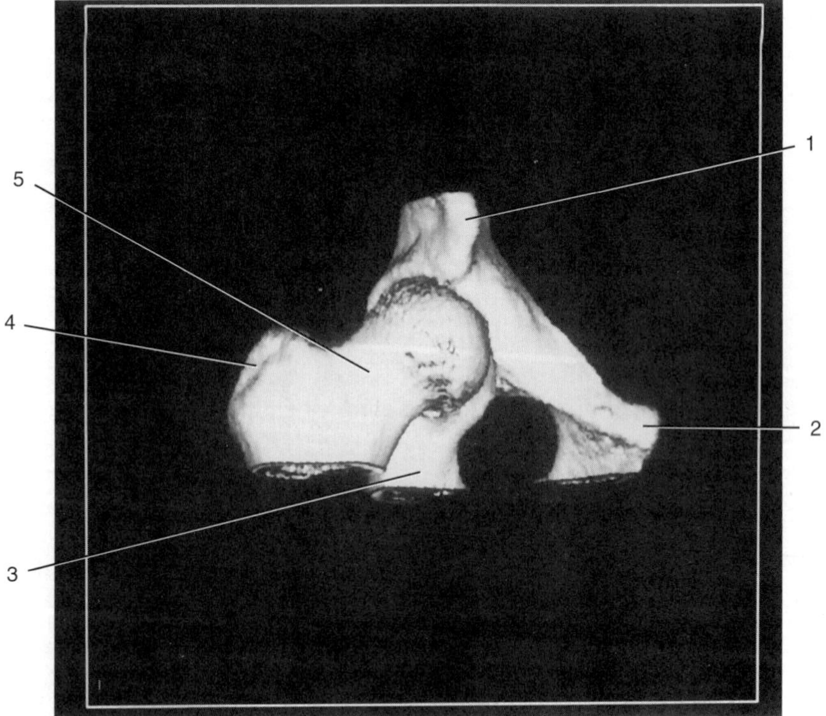

Figure 4–1.

34. Which of the following scan parameters should be used for a three-dimensional disarticulation study of the hip such as in the model shown?

1. 1- to 2-mm section width
2. small scan field of view (SFOV)
3. overlapping sections
   - a. 1 only
   - b. 1 and 2 only
   - c. 1 and 3 only
   - d. 1, 2, and 3

35. Number 1 corresponds to which of the following?

- a. ischium
- b. pubis
- c. ilium
- d. acetabulum

36. Number 5 corresponds to which of the following?

- a. sciatic notch
- b. humeral neck
- c. gluteal tuberosity
- d. femoral neck

37. Which of the following corresponds to the ischium?

- a. 1
- b. 4
- c. 2
- d. 3

38. Which of the following abnormal findings reduces the density of the liver?

- a. hyperdense cyst
- b. contrast-enhancing tumor
- c. fatty infiltrate
- d. all of the above

Questions 39–42 refer to Figure 4–2.

39. Which of the following corresponds to the retromandibular vein?
   a. 3
   b. 5
   c. 4
   d. none of the above

40. Which of the following sets of section widths and spacing is most suitable for a general survey CT of the neck?
   a. 1.5 mm thick every 1.5 mm
   b. 3 mm thick every 5 mm
   c. 5 mm thick every 5 mm
   d. 10 mm thick every 10 mm

41. Number 6 corresponds to which of the following?
   a. nasopharynx
   b. oropharynx
   c. esophagus
   d. larynx

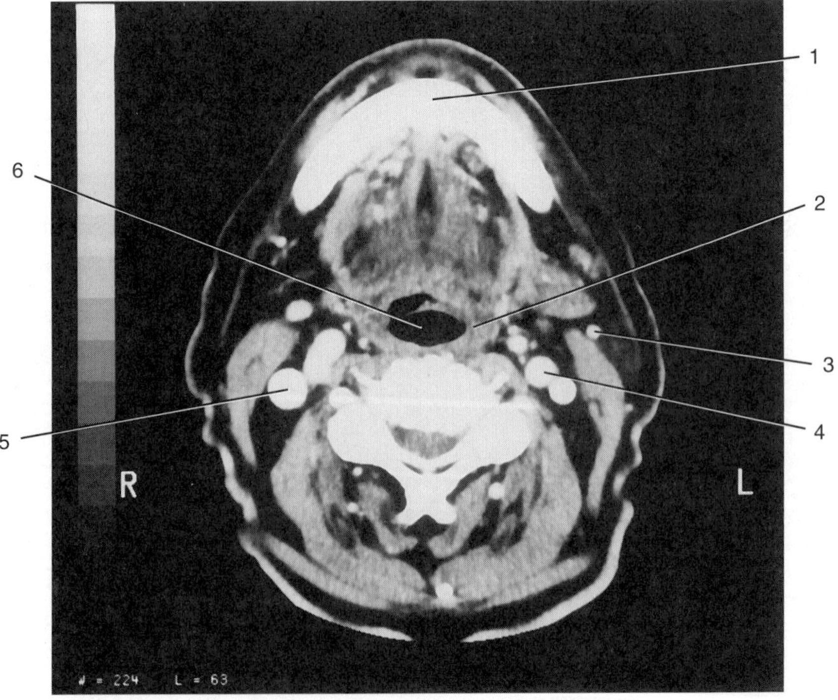

Figure 4–2.

42. Number 2 corresponds to which of the following?

a. adenoids
b. epiglottis
c. pharyngeal constrictor muscle
d. parotid gland

43. The ______________ gland is located in the anterosuperior portion of the mediastinum and is often identified with CT when scanning younger patients.

a. thyroid
b. Luschka
c. thymus
d. parathyroid

Questions 44–48 refer to Figure 4–3.

44. Number 6 corresponds to which of the following?
   a. round ligament
   b. longitudinal fissure
   c. falciform ligament
   d. transverse fissure

45. Number 5 corresponds to which of the following?
   a. right lobe of the liver
   b. quadrate lobe of the liver
   c. portal vein
   d. caudate lobe of the liver

46. Which of the following types of contrast media were administered to the patient for this CT examination of the abdomen?
   1. oral iodinated contrast
   2. oral effervescent negative contrast
   3. intravenous iodinated contrast
   a. 1 only
   b. 1 and 2 only
   c. 1 and 3 only
   d. 1, 2, and 3

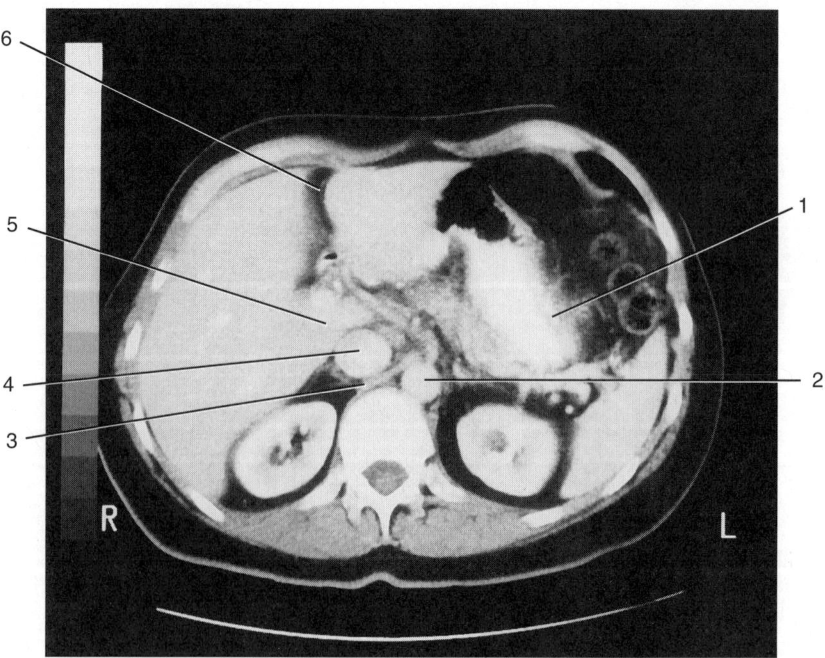

Figure 4–3.

47. Number 1 corresponds to which of the following?

a. gastric haustrae
b. digested food
c. gastric ulcers
d. gastric rugae

48. Number 3 corresponds to which of the following?

a. right renal vein
b. right crus of the diaphragm
c. right renal artery
d. superior mesenteric artery

49. Which of the following CT studies of the head may be performed without a contrast agent?

a. CT angiogram for the circle of Willis
b. coronal CT scan to rule out pituitary tumor
c. CT of the brain to rule out subdural hematoma
d. CT of the brain to rule out metastatic disease

Questions 50–52 refer to Figure 4–4.

50. Which of the following statements regarding the image is correct?

a. Oral iodinated contrast was administered 2 hours before scanning.

b. A small SFOV was used.

c. The width of the window used to display the image is approximately 2000 Hounsfield units.

d. The level of the window used to display the image is approximately −150 Hounsfield units.

51. Number 3 corresponds to which of the following?

a. vertebral foramen

b. pedicle

c. sacral canal

d. sacral foramen

52. Which of the following best describes the pathologic abnormality present?

a. metastatic disease of the sacrum

b. sacral cyst

c. fracture of the sacrum

d. dislocated sacroiliac joint

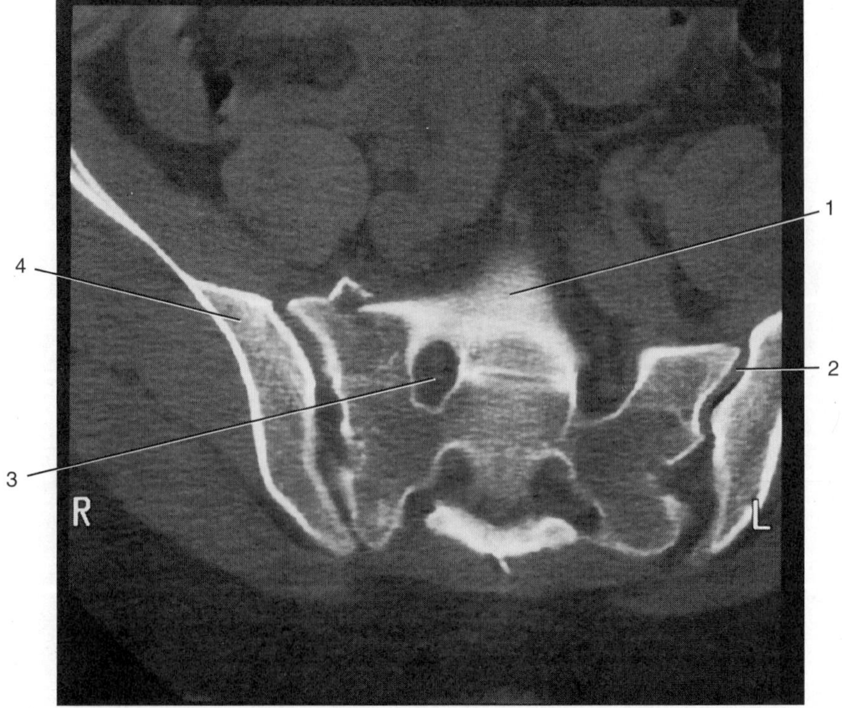

Figure 4–4.

53. CT scanning of the liver for tumor evaluation should not be performed during which of the following phases of contrast enhancement?

a. nonequilibrium phase
b. equilibrium phase
c. dynamic phase
d. bolus phase

54. The kidneys are usually located anatomically between which vertebrae?

a. T6 and L2
b. T12 and L3
c. L2 and L4
d. L3 and S1

Questions 55–59 refer to Figure 4–5.

55. Number 6 corresponds to which of the following?
   a. right brachiocephalic vein
   b. left subclavian artery
   c. brachiocephalic artery
   d. left common carotid artery

56. Number 2 corresponds to which of the following?
   a. right brachiocephalic vein
   b. left subclavian artery
   c. brachiocephalic artery
   d. left common carotid artery

57. Number 7 corresponds to which of the following?
   a. right brachiocephalic vein
   b. left subclavian artery
   c. brachiocephalic artery
   d. left common carotid artery

58. Which number corresponds to the left brachiocephalic vein?
   a. 2
   b. 4
   c. 5
   d. 1

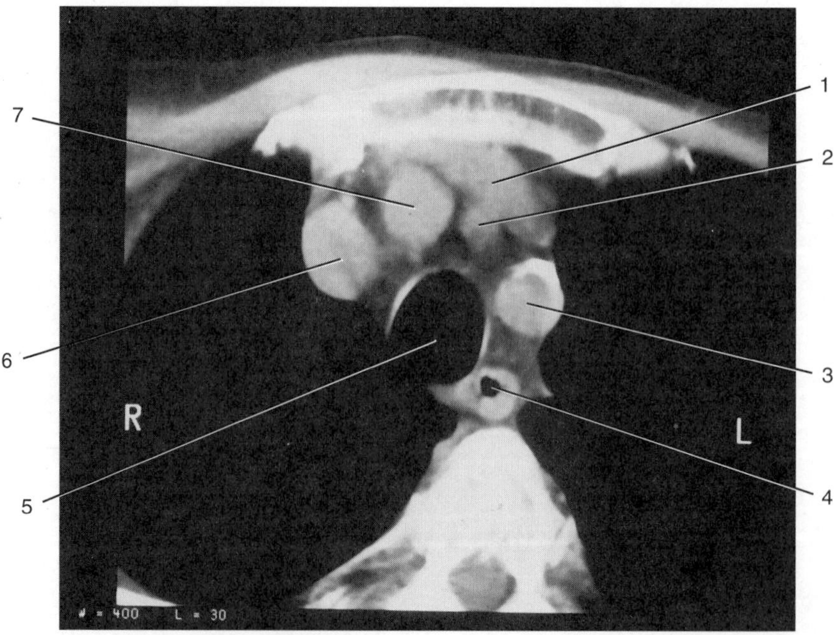

Figure 4–5.

59. Which of the following does not branch off from the aortic arch?

a. 6
b. 3
c. 7
d. 2

60. Axial CT images of the knee may be acquired in five separate series with knee flexions of 0°, 15°, 30°, 45°, and 60° in order to demonstrate the

a. tibial plateau
b. patellofemoral joint
c. medial and lateral menisci
d. anterior cruciate ligament

Questions 61–66 refer to Figure 4–6.

61. Number 5 corresponds to which of the following?
   a. right common iliac vein
   b. left common iliac vein
   c. right common iliac artery
   d. left common iliac artery

62. Number 4 corresponds to which of the following?
   a. erector spinae muscle
   b. sigmoid colon
   c. psoas muscle
   d. renal cyst

63. Number 3 corresponds to which of the following?
   a. anterior superior iliac spine
   b. iliac crest
   c. anterior inferior iliac spine
   d. spine of ischium

64. The vertebral body shown is most likely
   a. L2
   b. L3
   c. L4
   d. S1

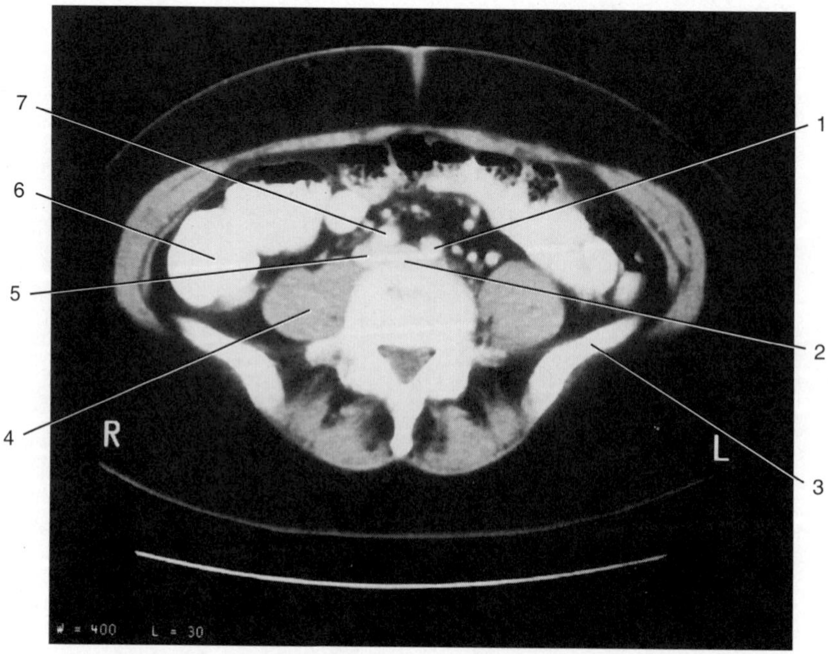

Figure 4–6.

65. Which of the following corresponds to the left common iliac artery?

a. 5
b. 2
c. 7
d. 1

66. Number 6 corresponds to which of the following?

a. descending colon
b. ileocecal valve
c. ascending colon
d. jejunum

Questions 67–72 refer to Figure 4–7.

67. Which of the following most accurately describes the position of the patient?
   a. prone with knees extended, feet dorsiflexed
   b. supine with knees flexed, plantar surface of feet resting on table
   c. supine with knees extended, feet hyperextended
   d. prone with knees flexed, feet hyperextended

68. Number 2 corresponds to which of the following?
   a. navicular
   b. cuboid
   c. cuneiform
   d. talus

69. Number 6 corresponds to which of the following?
   a. navicular
   b. cuboid
   c. cuneiform
   d. talus

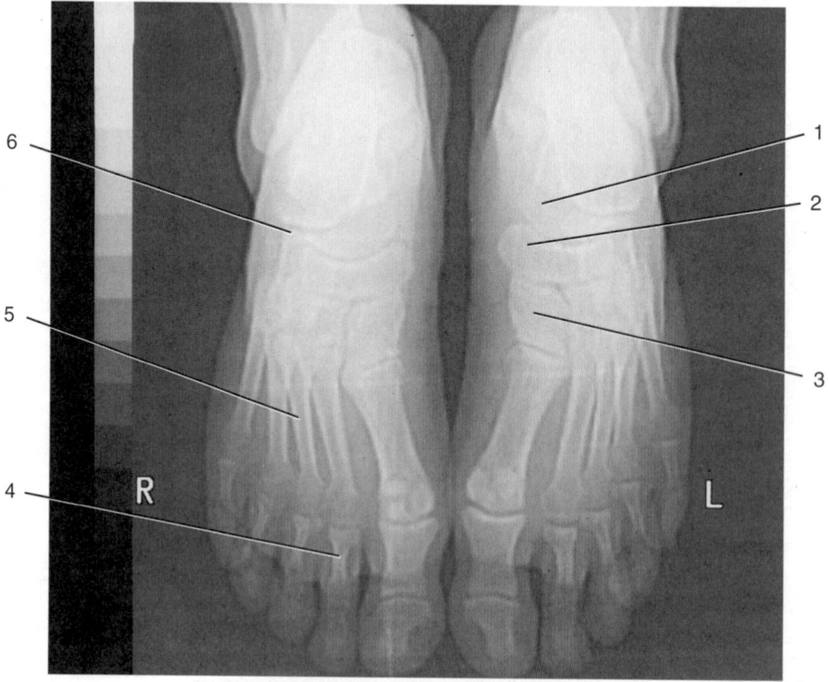

Figure 4–7.

70. Number 1 corresponds to which of the following?

a. cuboid
b. talus
c. calcaneus
d. navicular

71. Which of the following bones of the foot are included as tarsals?

1. third proximal phalanx
2. lateral cuneiform
3. first metatarsal

a. 1 only
b. 2 only
c. 2 and 3 only
d. 1, 2, and 3

72. CT images acquired in a plane perpendicular to the long axis of the scout image shown are considered ______________ images.

a. axial
b. sagittal
c. coronal
d. transaxial

73. A 15-second spiral CT scan of the pelvis is performed using a 1.0-cm aperture size. If a 1:1 pitch was used, the total length of coverage for this scan would be

a. 50 mm
b. 100 mm
c. 150 mm
d. 250 mm

Questions 74–79 refer to Figure 4–8.

74. Which of the following most accurately describes the proper position of the patient for a CT examination of the brain?
   a. prone with the head extended
   b. supine with the head extended
   c. prone with the chin down
   d. supine with the chin down

75. Number 4 corresponds to which of the following?
   a. fourth ventricle
   b. vein of Galen
   c. third ventricle
   d. thalamostriate vein

76. Number 3 corresponds to which of the following?
   a. cerebrum
   b. vermis of cerebellum
   c. tentorium cerebelli
   d. occipital lobe

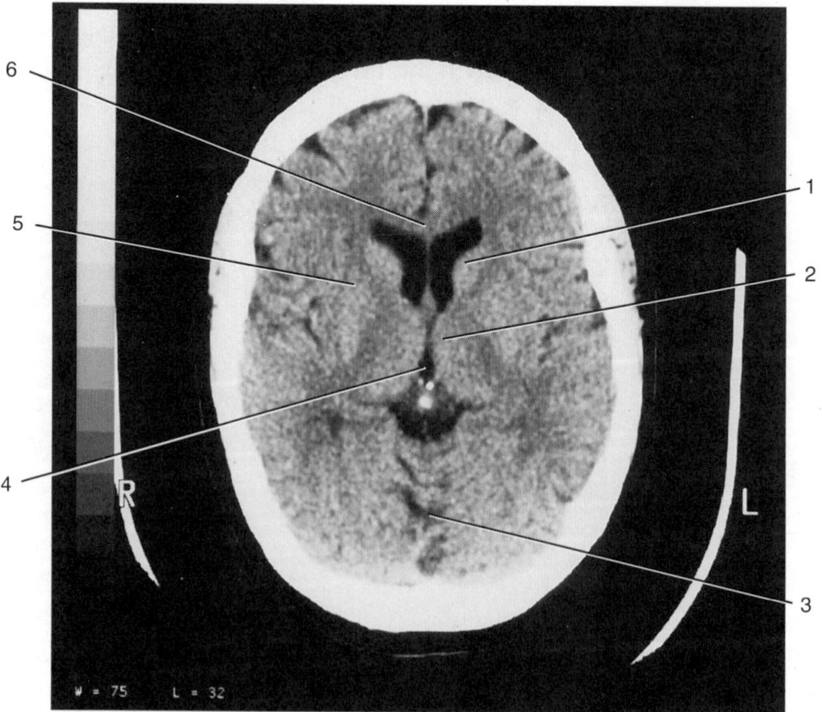

Figure 4–8.

77. Number 5 corresponds to which of the following?
   a. caudate nucleus
   b. putamen
   c. thalamus
   d. globus pallidus

78. Number 2 corresponds to which of the following?
   a. caudate nucleus
   b. putamen
   c. thalamus
   d. globus pallidus

79. Which of the following corresponds to the genu of corpus callosum?
   a. 6
   b. 5
   c. 2
   d. 1

80. A CT image should be viewed on the monitor in which of the following orientations?
   a. from the feet toward the head with the patient's left on the viewer's left
   b. from the feet toward the head with the patient's left on the viewer's right
   c. from the head toward the feet with the patient's right on the viewer's right
   d. from the head toward the feet with the patient's right on the viewer's left

81. In which of the following cranial nerves would an acoustic neuroma be found?
   a. third
   b. eighth
   c. tenth
   d. twelfth

Questions 82–86 refer to Figure 4–9.

82. Number 4 corresponds to which of the following?

a. spinous process
b. lamina
c. transverse process
d. pedicle

83. During a CT evaluation of a lumbar disk space, the scan range should include

a. from the midbody of the vertebra above to the midbody of the vertebra below
b. from below the spinous process of the vertebra above to just above the spinous process of the lower vertebra
c. the entire vertebral bodies both above and below the disk
d. from the pedicle of the vertebra above to the pedicle of the vertebra below

84. Which of the following corresponds to the pedicle?

a. 1
b. 4
c. 2
d. 3

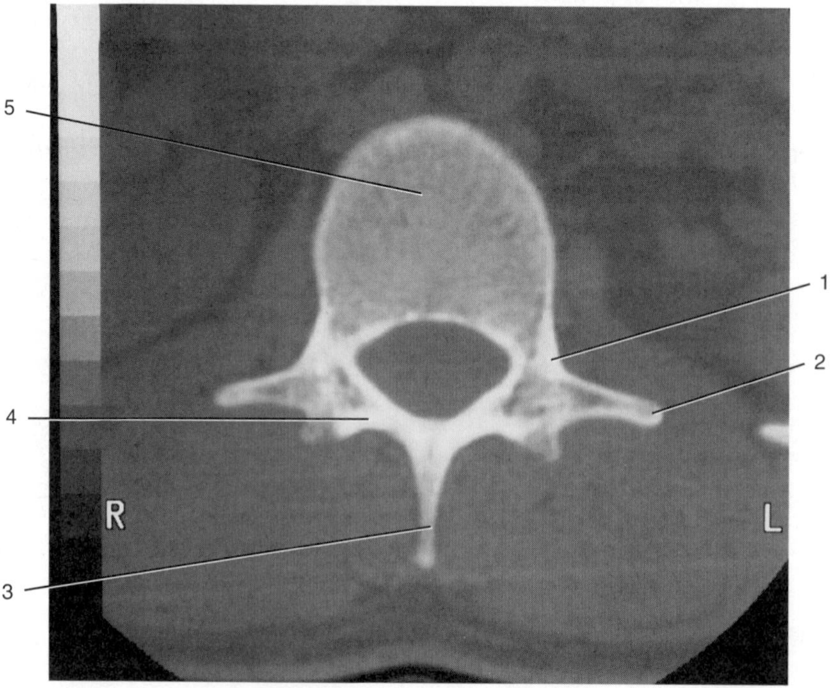

Figure 4–9.

85. The administration of intrathecal iodinated contrast in the patient shown in the figure would allow greater visualization of the

1. spinal cord
2. nerve roots
3. annulus fibrosis

   a. 1 only
   b. 1 and 2 only
   c. 1 and 3 only
   d. 1, 2, and 3

86. Number 3 corresponds to which of the following?

   a. pedicle
   b. transverse process
   c. lamina
   d. spinous process

87. Which of the following interscan delays would be used for a dynamic CT study of the chest?

   a. 4 seconds
   b. 8 seconds
   c. 12 seconds
   d. 15 seconds

Questions 88–90 refer to Figure 4–10.

88. The scout image shown could be used to prescribe a CT examination of the

a. chest
b. abdomen
c. thoracic spine
d. abdomen and pelvis

89. Some CT scanners enable the technologist to outline an anatomic area on a series of cross-sectional images and then define the outlined area on a scout or localizer image. This feature is called

a. treatment planning
b. density contouring
c. correlation
d. histogram

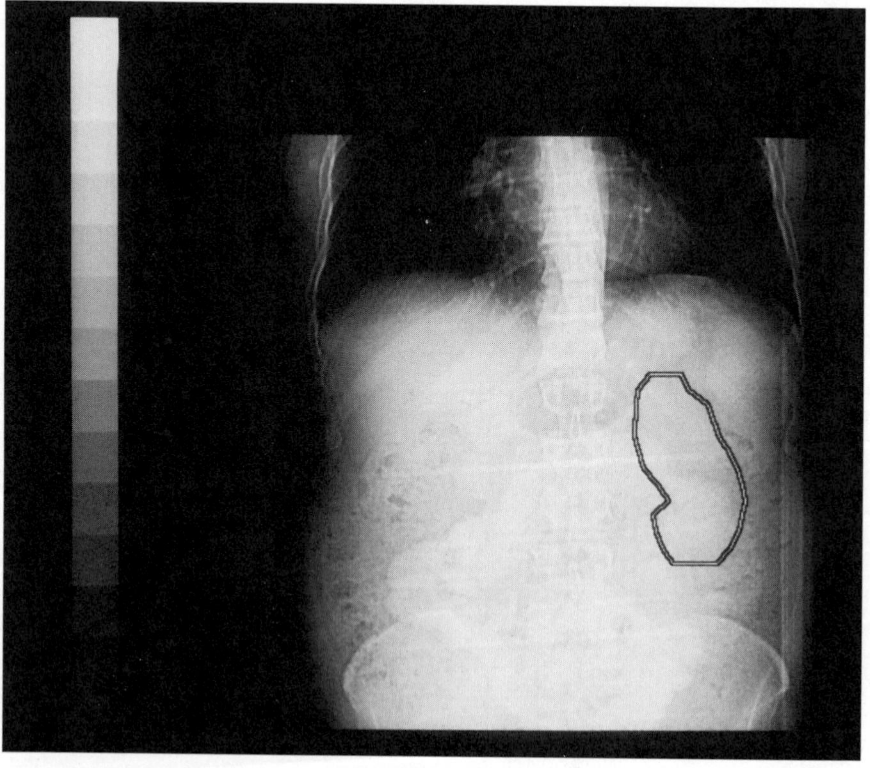

Figure 4–10.

90. The outlined area most likely represents the

a. stomach
b. left kidney
c. spleen
d. right kidney

Questions 91–95 refer to Figure 4–11.

91. Number 2 corresponds to which of the following?

a. right ventricle
b. right atrium
c. left ventricle
d. left atrium

92. Which of the following correctly lists the algorithm, matrix size, and section thickness used for this image?

a. soft tissue, 320, 5.0 mm
b. bone, 512, 10.0 mm
c. standard, 512, 5.0 mm
d. standard, 512, 10.0 mm

93. Number 4 corresponds to which of the following?

a. descending aorta
b. esophagus
c. azygos vein
d. trachea

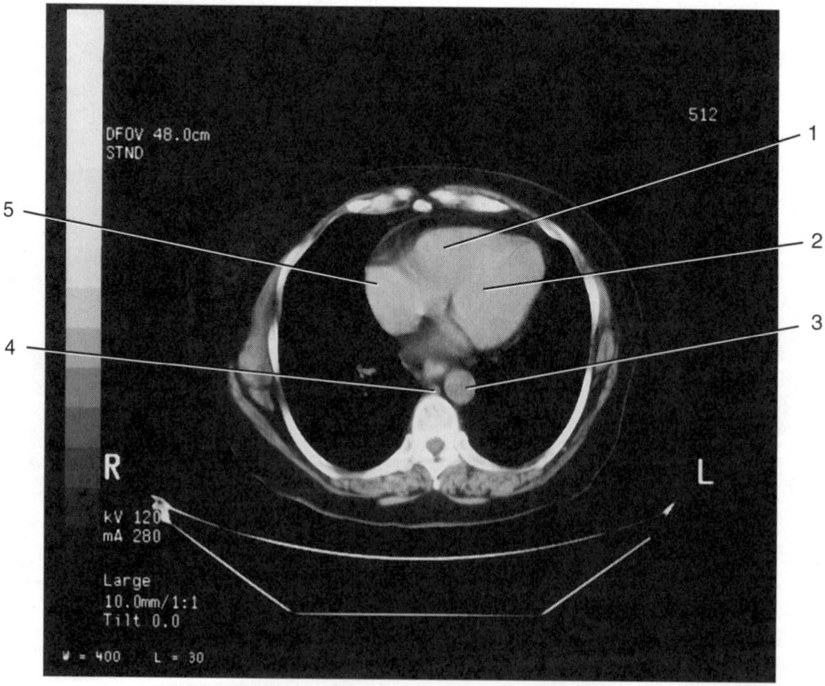

Figure 4–11.

94. Which of the following technical changes would improve the image quality?
   a. change of matrix size to 256
   b. decreased DFOV
   c. change of matrix size to 320
   d. increased DFOV

95. Which of the following corresponds to the left atrium?
   a. 2
   b. 5
   c. 1
   d. none of the above

96. Which of the following types of pathologic conditions cannot be easily diagnosed from a CT scan of the brain?
   a. astrocytoma
   b. traumatic hemorrhage
   c. cerebral infarct
   d. Alzheimer's disease

97. Most pancreatic tumors occur in the pancreatic
   a. head
   b. body
   c. tail
   d. uncinate process

Questions 98–101 refer to Figure 4–12.

98. Which number corresponds to the gluteus medius muscle?
  a. 5
  b. 7
  c. 2
  d. 3

99. Number 1 corresponds to which of the following?
  a. iliac vein
  b. femoral vein
  c. iliac artery
  d. femoral artery

100. Number 5 corresponds to which of the following?
  a. iliopsoas muscle
  b. sartorius muscle
  c. obturator internus muscle
  d. gluteus minimus muscle

101. Number 8 corresponds to which of the following?
  a. iliac vein
  b. femoral vein
  c. iliac artery
  d. femoral artery

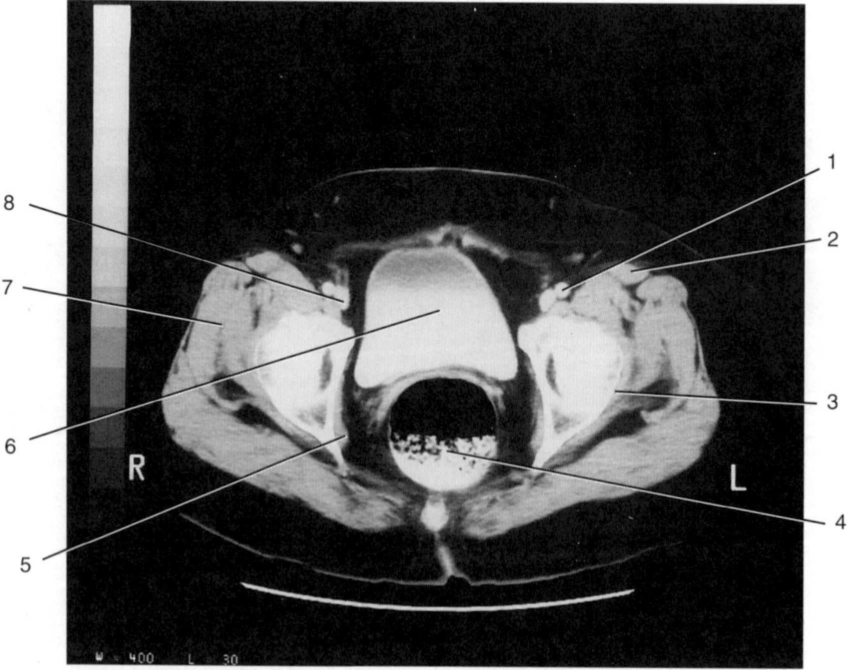

Figure 4–12.

102. Before scanning the liver after a bolus injection of iodinated contrast material, a delay of ______________ should be applied.

a. 0 seconds
b. 20 seconds
c. 45 seconds
d. 120 seconds

Questions 103–105 refer to Figure 4–13.

103. The type of image shown is referred to as a
  a. three-dimensional image
  b. retrospective image
  c. stereotactic image
  d. MPR image

104. Number 2 corresponds to which of the following?
  a. dental implants
  b. mandibular fractures
  c. surgical staples
  d. roots of teeth

105. Number 3 indicates that this image was generated from a series of ______________ CT images.
  a. sagittal
  b. axial
  c. coronal
  d. panoramic

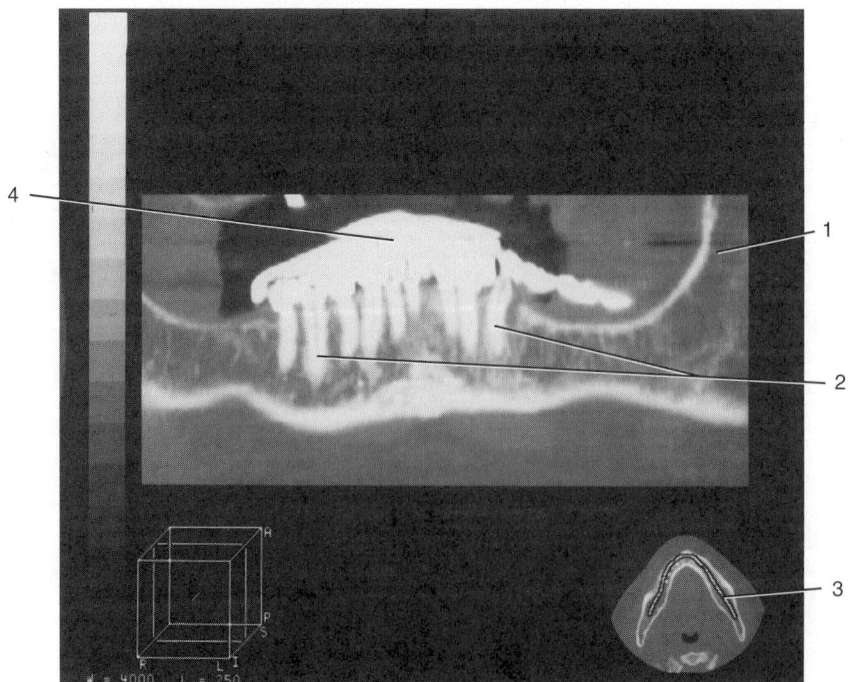

Figure 4–13.

C. Physics and Instrumentation

106. Which of the following technical changes may increase the partial volume effect present on a spiral CT scan?

a. decrease in pitch
b. decrease in aperture size
c. increase in matrix size
d. increase in pitch

107. During which of the following CT examinations is a misregistration artifact most likely to occur?

a. brain
b. pelvis
c. neck
d. abdomen

108. Which of the following mathematical functions may be used to quantify the spatial resolution of a CT scanner?

1. PSF
2. MTF
3. LSF

a. 2 only
b. 1 and 2 only
c. 2 and 3 only
d. 1, 2, and 3

109. The matrix size describes which of the following?

a. aperture size used during data acquisition
b. number of pixels used to display an image
c. relationship between the field of view and algorithm
d. none of the above

110. Which of the following is not an iterative method of CT image reconstruction?

a. point by point correction
b. Fourier transform
c. simultaneous reconstruction
d. ray by ray correction

111. The type of filter used at the x-ray tube of a CT scanner is called a

a. kernel
b. water bath
c. bow-tie filter
d. wedge filter

112. In the following formula used to calculate the linear attenuation coefficient, $I = I_0e^{-\mu x}$, the symbol I_0 identifies

a. Euler's constant
b. incident intensity
c. absorber thickness
d. transmitted intensity

113. Which of the following would increase the noise of a CT image?

a. increased mAs
b. decreased aperture size
c. decreased filtration
d. decreased matrix size

Questions 114–115 refer to Figure 4–14.

114. The technique that provides the detail of the outer portions of this three-dimensional model while maintaining the typical CT detail of the lungs inside is called

a. maximum intensity projection
b. surface rendering
c. summed projection
d. voxel gradient

115. Which of the following anatomic quadrants has been removed from the three-dimensional model?

a. left posterior inferior
b. right anterior inferior
c. left anterior superior
d. right anterior superior

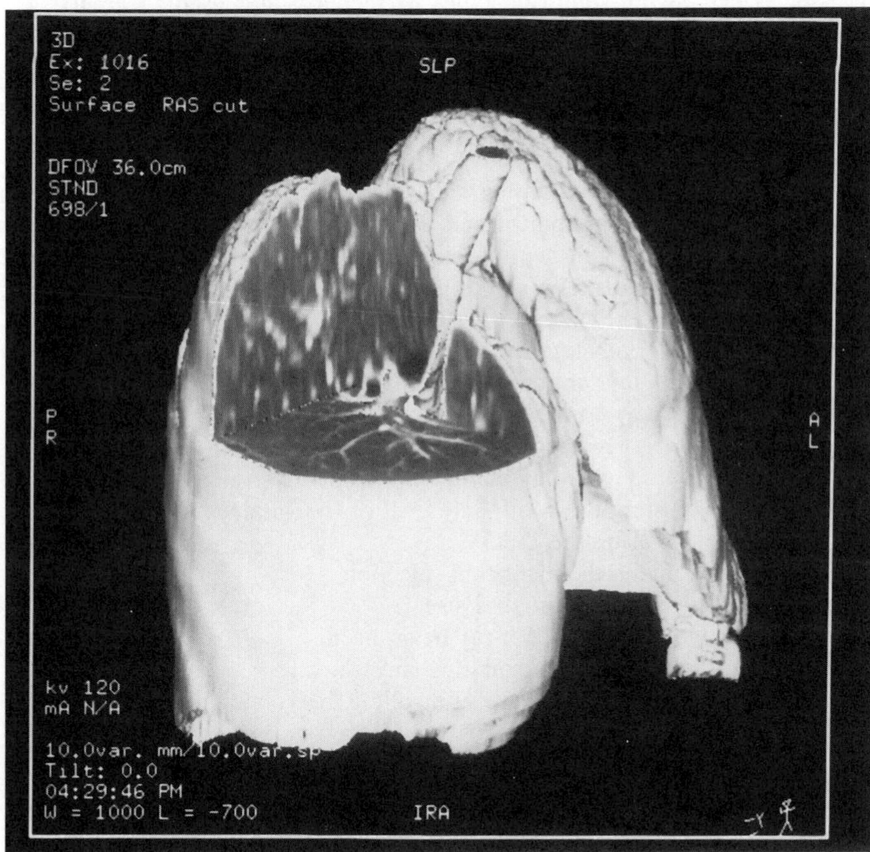

Figure 4–14.

116. The interaction between x-ray and matter that is responsible for the production of the scatter radiation absorbed by the patient and detectors is

a. Compton interaction
b. bremsstrahlung interaction
c. photoelectric effect
d. characteristic interaction

117. The types of detectors used in CT include

1. gas ionization
2. stimulable phosphor
3. scintillation crystal

a. 1 only
b. 3 only
c. 1 and 3 only
d. 2 and 3 only

118. Which of the following types of media is not used to archive CT images?

a. 3.5-inch floppy disk
b. magnetic tape
c. VHS tape
d. magnetic optical disk

119. A test phantom containing water is scanned, and five region of interest measurements are performed. The subsequent density measurements are compared and demonstrate a maximum deviation of less than 2 Hounsfield units. This quality assurance test was performed to evaluate the _______________ of the scanner.

a. spatial resolution
b. cross-field uniformity
c. signal-to-noise ratio
d. contrast resolution

120. Which of the following manipulations involve the use of image data?

a. adjusting the width and level of the window setting
b. decreasing the DFOV
c. changing the algorithm selection
d. increasing the matrix size

121. Collimation of the CT x-ray beam occurs

1. at the x-ray tube, regulating slice thickness
2. just prior to the patient, controlling the volume of tissue irradiated
3. prior to the detectors, limiting the amount of scatter radiation absorbed

a. 1 only
b. 1 and 2 only
c. 1 and 3 only
d. 1, 2, and 3

122. An average CT number value for bone is
   a. +100 Hounsfield units
   b. +500 Hounsfield units
   c. +1000 Hounsfield units
   d. +3000 Hounsfield units

123. A CT scanner capable of producing an image that is a perfect reproduction of the actual anatomic section is said to have an MTF of
   a. 0
   b. 1
   c. 10
   d. 100

124. The major disadvantage of the back-projection method of image reconstruction is the appearance of the
   a. partial volume effect
   b. ring artifact
   c. Gibbs phenomenon
   d. star artifact

125. Which of the following is used in gas ionization CT detectors?
   a. neon
   b. xenon
   c. helium
   d. nitrogen

126. The most effective method of reducing involuntary motion on a CT image is through
   a. immobilization
   b. thorough explanation of the examination to the patient
   c. reduced scan times
   d. physical restraint

127. Which of the following CT film formats provides the largest image for the viewer on a 14- × 17-inch film?
   a. 4:1
   b. 6:1
   c. 12:1
   d. 20:1

Questions 128–129 refer to Figure 4–15.

128. The circle deposited on the image is used to
- a. magnify a portion of the image
- b. localize an area for percutaneous biopsy
- c. perform a region of interest measurement
- d. produce an MPR image

129. The density measurement performed yielded an average CT number of zero. This area consists of
- a. fat
- b. blood
- c. water
- d. air

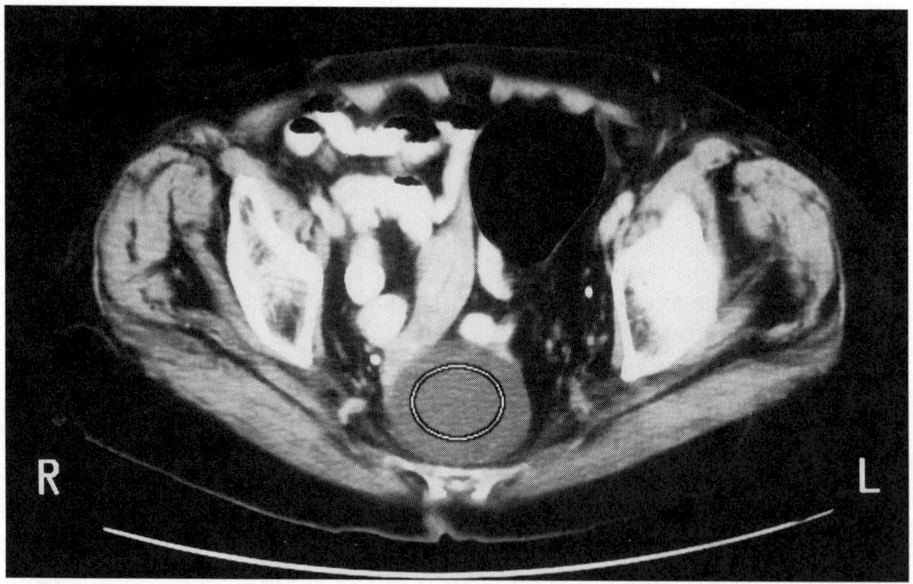

Figure 4–15.

130. Which of the following matrices provides the greatest spatial resolution?

a. 256 × 256
b. 320 × 320
c. 512 × 512
d. 1024 × 1024

131. The data acquisition system of a CT scanner

1. measures transmitted intensity
2. converts transmission data into a digital signal
3. sends the digital information to the central processing unit

a. 1 only
b. 2 only
c. 1 and 3 only
d. 1, 2, and 3

132. Which of the following terms is used to describe a set of rules for solving a mathematical problem?

a. reconstruction
b. algorithm
c. function
d. array

133. The contrast resolution of a CT scanner is not related to which of the following?

a. focal spot size
b. section width
c. reconstruction algorithm
d. signal-to-noise ratio

134. The spatial resolution of a CT scanner is usually expressed as

a. HU
b. lp/cm
c. μ
d. Hz

Questions 135–136 refer to Figure 4–16.

135. The processing technique used to include only bone tissue in this three-dimensional model of the pelvis is called
  a. voxel gradient
  b. maximum intensity projection
  c. thresholding
  d. summed projection

136. Which of the following would reduce the step artifact shown on the image?
  a. switch from standard algorithm to bone algorithm
  b. increase threshold setting
  c. reduce section width from 10 mm to 3 mm
  d. decrease threshold setting

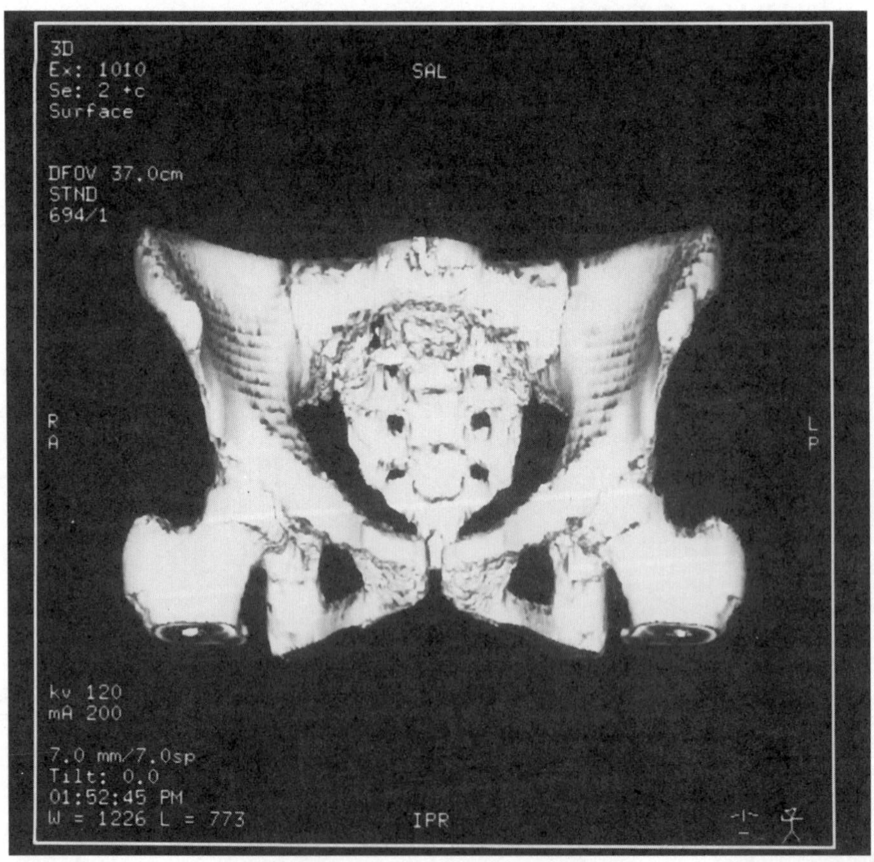

Figure 4–16.

137. When a SFOV is chosen, the CT technologist is controlling

a. the diameter of acquisition/reconstruction for the anatomic section
b. the number of activated detectors within the array
c. the correction factors for the specific area of anatomic interest
d. all of the above

138. A CT image is displayed in a window with a level of +200 and a width of 1000. Which of the following statements is correct?

a. Pixels with values between +200 and −1000 Hounsfield units appear white.
b. Pixels with values greater than +200 Hounsfield units appear black.
c. Pixels with values between −300 and +700 Hounsfield units are assigned shades of gray.
d. Pixels with values between −1200 and +1200 Hounsfield units are assigned shades of gray.

139. The dimension of a voxel may be decreased by which of the following?

a. decreasing the section width
b. decreasing the matrix size
c. increasing the section width
d. increasing the DFOV

140. A CT image of a homogeneous material contains variations in CT number from pixel to pixel. This image has

a. high contrast
b. sensitivity
c. definition
d. noise

141. Which of the following are correct statements concerning the translate–rotate mode of CT data acquisition?

1. Circular detector arrays of 360° are used.
2. Data are collected only during translation.
3. The method was used in first- and second-generation CT scanners.

a. 2 only
b. 3 only
c. 1 and 2 only
d. 2 and 3 only

142. As the attenuation of a volume of tissue decreases, the transmitted intensity of a CT x-ray beam

a. increases
b. remains unchanged
c. decreases
d. increases to a peak value and then rapidly decreases

143. Which of the following statements comparing the efficiency of scintillation and gas ionization detectors is correct?

a. Both have approximately the same capture efficiency.
b. The scintillation detector has a higher capture efficiency.
c. Unlike the scintillation detector, the gas ionization detector has a problem with afterglow.
d. Gas ionization detectors have a higher conversion efficiency.

144. Which of the following terms accurately describes the type of x-ray beam used in a third-generation CT scanner?

a. pencil beam
b. fan beam
c. nutating beam
d. electron beam

Question 145 refers to Figure 4–17.

145. The phantom image is used to test which of the following image quality factors of a CT scanner?

a. spatial resolution
b. noise
c. linearity
d. contrast resolution

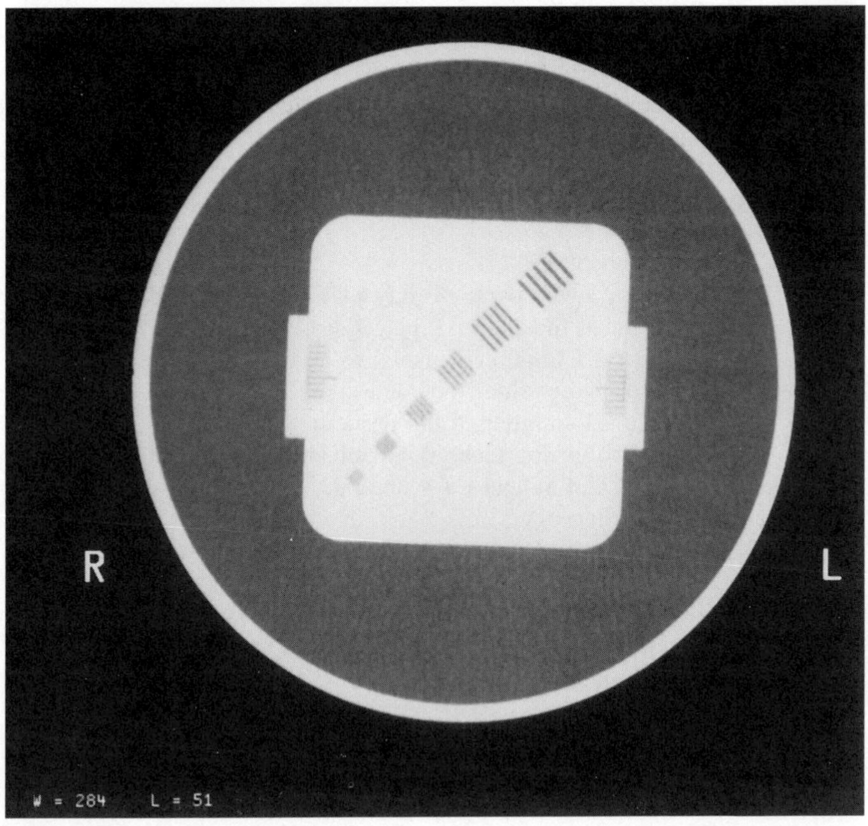

Figure 4–17.

146. Two adjacent pixels are measured to have a difference of 1 Hounsfield unit. This amounts to a tissue density difference of approximately

a. 0.1%
b. 1.0%
c. 10%
d. 25%

147. The intensity of the CT x-ray beam can be increased by

a. increasing filtration
b. decreasing collimation
c. decreasing applied tube voltage
d. increasing collimation

148. Which of the following is a solid-state device used to record the light flashes given off by a scintillation crystal?

a. photomultiplier tube
b. anode
c. photodiode
d. input phosphor

149. When choosing a window to display a CT image, the width defines the

a. midpoint of the range of pixels displayed
b. range of CT numbers (pixels) to be displayed
c. range of pixel values included in a region of interest
d. average CT number of the tissue of interest

150. Which of the following technologic advances has led to the development of spiral and helical CT scanning?

1. slip-ring technology
2. electron beam technology
3. high-efficiency x-ray tubes

a. 1 only
b. 1 and 2 only
c. 1 and 3 only
d. 1, 2, and 3

CHAPTER 5

Answer Key for Simulated Exam One

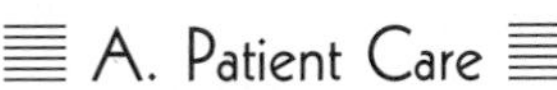

A. Patient Care

1. (b) The normal range for adult respirations is 12–20 breaths per minute. (Adler and Carlton, 1994, p.181)
2. (b) Parenteral administration involves the injection of medication into the body. Common routes of parenteral medication administration include intramuscular, intravenous, intradermal, and subcutaneous. (Ehrlich and McCloskey, 1989, p.124)
3. (a) Severe allergic reactions to iodinated intravenous contrast media can be reduced or eliminated with the administration of steroids or antihistamines before a CT examination. (Adler and Carlton, 1994, p.313)
4. (d) General signs and symptoms that a patient is going into shock include rapid breathing, tachycardia, hypotension, weak pulse, pallor, cyanosis, and cold, clammy skin. (Torres, 1993, p.91)
5. (b) Insertion of any intravenous line requires the use of sterile technique to prevent microorganisms from entering the bloodstream. (Adler and Carlton, 1994, p.235)
6. (d) Common sites for intravenous contrast injection include the antecubital, basilic, cephalic, and accessory cephalic veins. (Adler and Carlton, 1994, p.294)
7. (c) With no consideration for image quality, reductions in milliamperage (mA) or scan time (seconds) are direct methods of decreasing patient dose during a CT examination. (Seeram, 1994, p.227)
8. (d) The allergic history of a patient as well as present renal function status and cardiac illness history (e.g., high blood pressure, congestive heart failure) should always be discussed by the technologist or radi-

ologist before administration of any contrast material. (Adler and Carlton, 1994, p.313)

9. (b) Osmolality or osmotic concentration is the number of ions or particles formed when a substance (solute) dissociates in a given solution. It is described as the number of particles in solution per kilogram of water. (Adler and Carlton, 1994, p.310)
10. (d) The laboratory values blood urea nitrogen (BUN) and creatinine (a component of urine) can be used to indicate the status of a patient's renal function. (Adler and Carlton, 1994, p.314)
11. (b) During their stay within health care institutions, patients often acquire infections common to that institution. These infections are termed nosocomial. (Torres, 1993, p.23)
12. (a) Owing to the rotational nature of the x-ray tube, a patient receives exposure from all sides during a CT examination. Therefore, shields should be placed above and below the patient. (Seeram, 1994, p.306)
13. (d) Angiocatheters and lower-gauge needles are preferred for contrast administration with the use of a power injector. Being stable, an angiocatheter maintains proper placement within the vein while withstanding the high pressure applied by the power injector. (Chiu et al., 1995, p.84)
14. (b) Non-ionic contrast materials do not dissociate into charged particle (ions) when placed in solution. Ionic contrast materials are salts that form independent particles in aqueous solutions. (Carr, 1988, p.7)
15. (d) Good communication between the technologist and the patient is an extremely important factor in the production of high-quality CT examinations. Patients can be made to feel more comfortable, and when they are given detailed instructions, their increased cooperation can result in improved examination quality. (Chiu et al., 1995, p.11)
16. (c) The diameter of the lumen of a needle is known as its gauge. As the diameter of the lumen of a needle increases, its gauge decreases. (Torres, 1993, p.224)
17. (b) There are numerous factors that may be regarded as contraindications to iodinated contrast material administration. Two factors that increase the incidence of adverse reaction are multiple myeloma and prior severe reactions. (Torres, 1993, p.211)
18. (c) Checking the information located on the wristband is the most accurate method of verifying patient identification. (Adler and Carlton, 1994, p.286)
19. (c) Adjustable flow rate automatic injectors improve overall enhancement levels and offer consistency throughout an examination and between individual patients. (Seeram, 1994, p.295)
20. (b) The average range for normal adult blood urea nitrogen (BUN) levels is approximately 5–20 mg/dL. (*Mosby's Medical Dictionary*, 1994, Appendix A)

21. (a) The term vasovagal pertains to systemic hypotension often leading to cerebral ischemia. (*Mosby's Medical Dictionary*, 1994)
22. (d) During the photoelectric interaction, the object (patient) completely absorbs the energy of the incident x-ray photon. This results in an increase in dose as compared with scattering interactions. (Curry et al., 1990, p.62)
23. (c) Examples of mild adverse reactions to iodinated contrast material include nausea, mild urticaria, and a warm flushed sensation. Dyspnea, or difficulty breathing, is a moderate reaction. (Putman and Ravin, 1994, p.1068)
24. (d) The patient is required to provide informed consent before the start of any invasive procedure. The administration of intravascular contrast material is invasive and does require the informed consent of the patient. (Adler and Carlton, 1994, p.350)
25. (a) Chloral hydrate is an effective and commonly used sedative for children undergoing CT studies. (Adler and Carlton, 1994, p.285)
26. (d) Diatrizoate, iothalamate, and metrizoate are the generic names for three of the basic types of iodinated contrast media. They are more commonly known by their trade names, Hypaque, Conray, and Isopaque, respectively. (Carr, 1988, p.7)
27. (b) The categories of isolation technique are drainage–secretion precautions, enteric precautions, acid-fast bacillus isolation, respiratory isolation, contact isolation, and strict isolation. (Torres, 1993, p.38)
28. (c) Non-ionic iodinated contrast media have a lower osmolality and a lower incidence of adverse reaction in comparison with ionic contrast media. Both types of materials contain iodine in various concentrations. (Putman and Ravin, 1994, p.1069)
29. (b) A bolus injection is one in which the entire volume of medication or contrast is administered at once over a short period of time. (*Mosby's Medical Dictionary,* 1994)
30. (a) Intrathecal injections of iodinated contrast material are typically used in the CT evaluation of the lumbar spine. This type of injection introduces contrast directly into the subarachnoid space, which is located between the arachnoid and pia mater. The subarachnoid space contains the cerebrospinal fluid. (Chiu et al., 1995, p.162)

B. Imaging Procedures

31. (c) Contrast enhancement greatly improves demonstration of lymphadenopathy within the chest when compared with other mediastinal structures. (Seeram, 1994, p.280)
32. (a) Thin sections are required to assess abnormalities of the minute structures of the inner ear properly. The thinnest sections possible will provide maximum detail. (Seeram, 1994, p.269)

33. (d) The small bowel consists of three portions: the duodenum, the jejunum, and the ileum. The cecum is the proximal portion of the large bowel and is connected to the small bowel at the ileocecal valve. (Clemente, 1985, p.1469)
34. (b) For best demonstration of lumbar vertebral disk spaces, the plane of imaging should be parallel to the plane of the disk spaces. (Seeram, 1994, p.270)
35. (b) Inferior vena cava (Bo et al., 1990, p.126)
36. (a) Spleen (Bo et al., 1990, p.130)
37. (c) Patients with histories of headaches or dizziness should be evaluated for abnormalities of the inner ear. Thin sections (5 mm) through the posterior fossa are required to best demonstrate the small anatomic structures and improve image quality. (Seeram, 1994, p.269)
38. (d) A hemangioma is a congenital, benign mass containing blood-filled spaces. They are commonly found in the liver and spleen. (*Mosby's Medical Dictionary*, 1994)
39. (b) Simple cysts contain primarily water and therefore exhibit CT numbers ranging from approximately 0 (or slightly below) to +20 Hounsfield units. (Seeram, 1994, p.235)
40. (a) Left ovary (Chiu et al., 1995, p.156)
41. (d) Uterus (Chiu et al., 1995, p.156)
42. (b) Bladder (Chiu et al., 1995, p.156)
43. (d) The scan field of view (SFOV) chosen must be larger than the width of the patient to eliminate out-of-field artifacts. Some CT scanners may have limited choices for SFOVs. Other common terms include full-field, half-field, body-cal, and head-cal. (Berland, 1987, p.46)
44. (a) Patient inspiration provides optimal chest expansion and allows for improved demonstration of anatomic structures. (Berland, 1987, p.223)
45. (c) Three-dimensional studies are best performed using narrow sections acquired with no spacing, or preferably with an overlap, and a detail (bone) algorithm when imaging bony structures. (Seeram, 1994, p.252)
46. (d) CT examinations of the chest usually require that the patient be placed in the supine position. Patients may also be scanned prone to increase aeration of the posterior lung base, or they may be scanned in lateral decubitus positions to help differentiate certain types of pathologic conditions. (Moss et al., 1992, p.12)
47. (d) Spiral or helical CT examinations are obtained with the scanner continuously acquiring data as the patient travels through the gantry. The data acquired are volumetric in that they contain all of the attenuation information for a given area of anatomy. (Seeram, 1994, p.110)
48. (b) Right ventricle (Bo et al., 1990, p.102)
49. (b) Number 2 corresponds to the left atrium. (Bo et al., 1990, p.102)

50. (a) Azygos vein (Bo et al., 1990, p.102)
51. (d) Narrow sections (3 mm, 5 mm) are required in both the axial and coronal planes to properly demonstrate the orbits. (Seeram, 1994, p.269)
52. (c) Dynamic CT studies involve the use of a rapid bolus injection of contrast material accompanied by immediate, continuous scanning with the shortest interscan delays possible. (Seeram, 1994, p.295)
53. (d) Opacification of the stomach and bowel loops is imperative when scanning the abdomen and pelvis. Effervescent agents may be used to ensure proper gastric distension. Intravenous contrast agents are used to opacify blood vessels and are helpful in anatomic differentiation and evaluation of mass vascularity. (Seeram, 1994, p. 294)
54. (b) Number 5 corresponds to the anterior horn of the lateral ventricle. (Bo et al, 1990, p.12)
55. (b) Thalamus (Bo et al., 1990, p.12)
56. (c) Number 4 corresponds to the septum pellucidum. (Bo et al., 1990, p.12)
57. (c) The chest is most completely evaluated for bronchogenic carcinoma with sections performed from the apices through the liver. The adrenal gland and liver are common sites for metastatic disease in patients with primary lung neoplasm. Scanning may be done in a caudocranial direction to ensure maximum contrast enhancement of the liver and adrenals where indicated. (Moss et al., 1992, p.188)
58. (b) A total of 400–600 mL of oral contrast administered 45–90 minutes before the examination should opacify the small bowel, while the administration of additional contrast (300 mL) immediately before the examination should ensure gastric opacification. Administration of contrast via enema is indicated when evaluating the distal large bowel. (Seeram, 1994, p.294)
59. (c) A lateral projection of the head from below the skull base through the vertex is used as a scout (scanogram) for a CT scan of the brain. (Chiu et al., 1995, p.21)
60. (d) Number 6 corresponds to cholelithiasis, or the presence of gallstones in the bladder. This type of dense stone is well delineated on the CT image. Other types of radiolucent and isodense stones are not imaged as well with CT. (Moss et al., 1992, p.842)
61. (c) Number 1 corresponds to the superior mesenteric vein; it appears larger than the superior mesenteric artery, which is located just posterior to the vein. (Barrett et al., 1994, p.86)
62. (a) The duodenum is easily differentiated from the pancreatic head with the administration of oral contrast. (Bo et al., 1990, p.134)
63. (c) The window setting used to display this abdominal image uses a level of +50 and a width of +400. This is within the range of window settings commonly used to display images of the abdomen, pelvis, and

other predominantly soft-tissue structures. The level is set at a value near the average attenuation of the tissues of interest. A width of 400 is relatively narrow and is used to demonstrate various soft-tissue structures having similar densities. (Seeram, 1994, p.167)

64. (d) The glomerulus is the portion of the nephron that filters unwanted substances from blood plasma. The blood enters into the glomerulus through the afferent arteriole and exits through the efferent arteriole. The waste fluid leaves the glomerulus through the proximal tubule. (Guyton, 1986, p.393)
65. (b) The spinal cord extends to the lower margin of the first lumbar vertebra or to the upper margin of the second lumbar vertebra. At this level, it tapers to a point, known as the conus medullaris. (Clemente, 1985, p.959)
66. (a) Complete CT scans of the pelvis should range from the iliac crests to the pubic symphysis. This scan range may be extended if warranted. Scan parameters (i.e., slice thickness, incrementation) can be adjusted to correlate with the clinical history of the patient. (Berland, 1987, p.239)
67. (b) Iodinated intravenous contrast alters the CT image by increasing the density of enhanced structures. Organs and blood vessels containing iodine attenuate a greater portion of the primary beam, thereby increasing their attenuation value. This permits greater differentiation of anatomic structures and pathologic processes. Any "enhanced" structure has an increased attenuation value (and subsequent image density) when compared with normal, unenhanced structures. (Seeram, 1994, p.271)
68. (b) The pituitary and other structures involving the sella turcica are usually imaged in the coronal plane with CT. The coronal plane provides the best visualization of the pituitary gland with regard to its position within the sella turcica and reduces partial volume averaging of the pituitary with surrounding structures when compared with scans obtained in the axial plane. (Chiu et al., 1995, p.37)
69. (b) Number 2 corresponds to the lamina. (Wicke, 1994, p.236)
70. (c) The cauda equina is the extension of the spinal cord beyond its neural termination at the L1–L2 level. It consists of a collection of rootlets extending inferior from the conus medullaris. (Wicke, 1994, p.236)
71. (b) CT examination of the lumbar spine should be performed with narrow sections obtained parallel to the disk spaces with standard (soft tissue) algorithm selection to demonstrate the spinal cord and intervertebral disk material. (Seeram, 1994, p.270)
72. (b) Most mature spermatozoa are stored in the vas deferens. Spermatozoa are produced in the seminiferous tubules and pass through

the epididymis, where a small amount may also be stored. (Guyton, 1986, p.956)

73. (d) The patient should be instructed to phonate the letter "E" during CT scanning of the larynx. As data are acquired during scanning, the patient's phonation requires vibration of the vocal cords, thus allowing for thorough evaluation of their mobility. (Berland, 1987, p.216)
74. (c) Peristalsis is the rhythmic contraction of smooth muscle that propels material through the gastrointestinal tract. It is also commonly found in the bile duct and ureters. (Guyton, 1986, p.758)
75. (a) The frontal sinuses are absent at birth and do not usually fully develop until after puberty. The ethmoidal, maxillary, and sphenoidal sinuses begin to develop during gestation. (Clemente, 1985, p.1364)
76. (b) CT scans are commonly performed for radiation therapy treatment planning. The purpose of the examination is to precisely locate the area of interest for therapeutic treatment with radiation. It is important that the patient position during the CT examination be exactly the same as that which is used during radiation therapy treatment. To achieve this positioning, a flat tabletop produced with a board or foam insert is used. Equally important is the display field of view (DFOV) chosen by the technologist. It must be large enough to include the entire surface of the anatomic part. (Berland, 1987, p.244)
77. (a) Left pulmonary artery (Bo et al., 1990, p.86)
78. (a) Number 4 corresponds to the superior vena cava (Bo et al., 1990, p.86)
79. (d) Pleural effusions are commonly seen in the posterior portion of the lung field with the patient in a supine position on the CT table. Differentiation between pleural effusion and pleural thickening is made when region of interest measurements reveal fluid with density readings that are zero or slightly more than zero. Pleural effusion may be caused by multiple pathologic processes including infection, neoplasm, and congestive heart failure. (Moss et al., 1992, p.264)
80. (c) The third and fourth ventricles communicate through the cerebral aqueduct, which is commonly referred to as the aqueduct of Sylvius. (Clemente, 1985, p.1034)
81. (b) The duodenum and pancreatic head are often difficult to distinguish. This is one important reason why the small bowel must be properly opacified. To accomplish adequate opacification, oral contrast should be administered at least 30 minutes before scanning. Positioning the patient in a right lateral decubitus position is also helpful in ensuring opacification of the duodenum, which surrounds the pancreatic head. (Putman and Ravin, 1994, p.990)
82. (c) The term glioma refers to the group of glial tumors that occur in the brain. Glial cells are connective neural cells that play a supportive

role in the brain. There are several common types of gliomas, including astrocytomas and glioblastomas. (Putman and Ravin, 1994, p.206)

83. (a) Excretion half-time is a value describing the amount of time necessary for 50% of the contrast administered to be filtered by the renal system. In patients with normal renal function, the half-time is usually between 1 and 2 hours. (Katzberg, 1992, p. 8)
84. (d) The midcoronal plane passes through the body vertically, dividing it into equal anterior and posterior portions. The midsagittal plane divides the body into equal right and left portions. Any axial (transverse, horizontal) plane is one occurring at right angles to the coronal and sagittal planes and divides the body into superior and inferior portions. (Clemente, 1985, p.2)
85. (b) The term azotemia describes the condition of excessive nitrogenous materials in the blood. This condition is also commonly called uremia. Azotemia is a symptom of renal insufficiency and may occur during chronic renal failure. (Copstead, 1995, p.590)
86. (c) Dosage calculations for intravenous contrast administration in the pediatric patient are usually made following the general rule of 1 mL per pound of body weight. (Katzberg, 1992, p.211)
87. (d) The paranasal sinuses are best demonstrated by CT examination with images acquired in both the axial and the coronal plane. (Seeram, 1994, p.269)
88. (a) Nasopharynx (Bo et al., 1990, p.28)
89. (a) Number 4 corresponds to the right lateral pterygoid plate. (Bo et al., 1990, p.28)
90. (b) The nasal septum is a cartilaginous process that vertically separates the nasal cavities. The nasal septum in the figure deviates, or abnormally curves, toward the left. (Clemente, 1985, p.173)
91. (b) Contiguous acquisition with narrow slice thickness is preferred during CT examination of the cervical spine. Sections 3 mm thick or smaller should be used with no gap or even an overlap, thus ensuring thorough evaluation of the relatively small intervertebral disk spaces. (Seeram, 1994, p.270)
92. (c) Following intravenous contrast administration, three phases of enhancement occur: bolus phase, nonequilibrium phase, and equilibrium phase. The bolus phase occurs first, immediately after the bolus administration of contrast. The nonequilibrium phase is next, followed lastly by the equilibrium phase. During CT examination of the liver, scanning must occur during the first two phases of enhancement. It is possible for hepatic tumors to become isodense with surrounding tissue during the equilibrium phase, thereby limiting their visualization. (Katzberg, 1992, p.68)
93. (c) The mediastinum is a potential space located between the two lungs. It contains the heart, great blood vessels, thymus, and portions of the trachea and esophagus. (Clemente, 1985, p.1383)

94. (d) A coronal scout (or pilot) projection of the head may be obtained with the patient in either the supine or prone position. In the supine position, patients hyperextend the neck by dropping the head back so that it rests on its vertex on a positioning support device. In the prone position, patients extend the neck with the head resting on the chin. Coronal CT images may be produced in either case with the imaging plane positioned parallel to the coronal plane of the patient's head. (Chiu et al., 1995, p.37)
95. (d) Posterior clinoid process (Wicke, 1994, p.4)
96. (a) External auditory meatus (Wicke, 1994, p.4)
97. (d) The lateral projection of the head with the patient in the prone or supine position may be used as a localizer for all CT studies requiring coronal sections. Types of CT studies requiring coronal sections include those of the paranasal sinuses, pituitary gland, internal auditory canals, temporal bones, temporomandibular joints, and orbits and facial bones. (Seeram, 1994, p.269)
98. (c) The administration of intravenous contrast is not necessary to rule out a possible fracture during CT evaluation of an extremity. However, the use of narrow sections, bone windows, and bilateral scans is helpful in demonstrating this type of condition. (Seeram, 1994, p.299)
99. (b) The range of 1.0–3.0 mL/sec should be sufficient to provide the enhancement necessary for proper evaluation of the abdomen. This is a general range and may be adjusted to meet the needs of the examination at the discretion of the physician and medical personnel involved. (Katzberg, 1992, p.78)
100. (c) CT is commonly used during percutaneous aspiration and drainage procedures. CT images allow the radiologist to view the precise location of abnormal fluid collections and allow for accurate planning of a safe access route for the aspiration procedure. CT-guided aspiration of an abdominal abscess can be a valuable nonsurgical therapeutic technique. This type of procedure can also be used to reduce other types of abnormal fluid collections including cysts, bilomas, urinomas, and lymphoceles. (Lee et al., 1989, p.99)
101. (a) Positive contrast can be administered into the large bowel via enema to achieve thorough opacification. A dose of 150–250 mL should be sufficient to opacify the rectosigmoid region. Doses of 300–500 mL may be necessary to opacify the large bowel in its entirety. (Katzberg, 1992, p.204)
102. (b) Owing to its location and attenuation value, this structure is most likely an ovarian cyst. This cyst is present on the right ovary and has an attenuation value of +10. Cysts of the ovary, as well as those occurring elsewhere in the body, have attenuation values close to that of water or near zero. (Moss et al., 1992, p.1219)
103. (c) Uterus (Bo et al., 1990, p.246)

104. (d) Psoas major muscle (Bo et al., 1990, p.246)
105. (b) Number 6 corresponds to the ilium. (Bo et al., 1990, p.246)

C. Physics and Instrumentation

106. (d) Partial volume averaging of the CT image can be reduced by either slightly adjusting the slice location or reducing the slice thickness. A change in matrix size does not significantly alter the partial volume effect. (Berland, 1987, p.160)
107. (b) Misregistration is an artifact that occurs when a patient suspends respiration at different depths during consecutive scans. It results in the loss of anatomic information. (Berland, 1987, p.169)
108. (c) The back-projection method of image reconstruction involves the acquisition of attenuation values that are then projected back onto a matrix for subsequent display. (Seeram, 1994, p.130)
109. (d) The dimension of a pixel may be calculated by dividing the field of view by the matrix size. The DFOV of 25.6 cm must first be converted to 256 mm. This is then divided by 512 mm for a pixel dimension of 0.5 mm. The pixel is a two-dimensional item, square in shape, and the measurement of 0.5 mm corresponds to only one side. The numeric lengths of 0.5 mm and 0.05 cm are equal. (Seeram, 1994, p.79)
110. (b) The Lambert-Beer law, $I = I_0e^{-\mu x}$, is used to calculate the attenuation coefficient of a volume of material, where x equals the thickness of the absorber attenuating the radiation. (Seeram, 1994, p.104)
111. (c) First-generation CT scanners acquired data through a process based on a principle of tube translation and rotation around a patient's head. (Seeram, 1994, p.88)
112. (a) The CT number is based on the attenuation value of a voxel of tissue. The Hounsfield unit is the current unit used for this value. (Berland, 1987, p.93)
113. (b) Magnetic tape and magnetic optical disk are two commonly used media for CT image archival. (Seeram, 1994, p.14)
114. (b) Attenuation is the reduction in intensity of an x-ray beam as it interacts with matter. There are several interactions that cause attenuation of primary radiation, including Compton scatter and photoelectric effect. Each of these interactions reduces the energy or number of x-ray photons in a primary beam. (Curry et al., 1990, p.70)
115. (b) The use of a fan-shaped x-ray beam during CT imaging increases the total volume of tissue irradiated, thereby increasing the amount of scatter radiation produced. This significantly increases patient dose when compared with the "pencil beam" radiation used in older CT scanners. (Curry et al., 1990, p.296)
116. (a) The most common cause of CT image noise is the fluctuation in the number of x-ray photons measured by the detectors. When a CT scanner attempts to reconstruct an image from an insufficient amount

of transmitted radiation measurements, "statistical noise" occurs. (Curry et al., 1990, p.311)

117. (c) Scintillation crystals are used for all rotate–fixed (fourth-generation) CT scanners. The rotate–fixed geometry causes the relationship between the tube and the detectors to change continuously. A detector with a high intrinsic efficiency is necessary to improve the measurement of transmission information incident upon each detector. Information can be obscured when photons are measured by a detector and then are measured by another detector. Known as "detector crosstalk," this situation can be averted with the use of scintillation detectors in fourth-generation CT scanners. (Curry et al., 1990, p.299)
118. (c) First-generation CT scanners were based on a translate–rotate principle. The x-ray tube and detectors translate across the patient's head and then rotate 1°. This process repeats in a semicircular fashion, for 180° around the patient's head. (Seeram, 1994, p.88)
119. (c) The dimension of a voxel is determined by multiplying the pixel dimension by the slice thickness. The pixel dimension is directly controlled by the matrix size and the field of view. (Seeram, 1994, p.80)
120. (b) The contrast of a CT image is controlled by the spatial frequencies of the tissues within the section. Tissues of differing densities are represented electronically by different spatial frequencies. Adjacent tissues that greatly differ in density are represented by high spatial frequencies. (Berland, 1987, p.33)
121. (c) The operator may control the contrast and brightness of the CT image by adjusting the "window" setting. As a form of gray-scale mapping, the window determines the pixels assigned shades of gray based on their CT number. (Seeram, 1994, p.166)
122. (c) The analytic methods of CT image reconstruction include the filtered back-projection and the Fourier transform method. These techniques are called analytic because they use precise formulas for image reconstruction. (Curry et al., 1990, p.306)
123. (d) The magnetic optical disk is capable of storing approximately 1500 512^2 matrix CT images. This is considerably more than magnetic tape, which was previously the standard choice for CT image archival. (Seeram, 1994, p.153)
124. (a) Linearity describes the relationship between the CT number and actual linear attenuation coefficients of an object. It is used to measure the accuracy of a CT scanner. (Seeram, 1994, p.211)
125. (d) The array processor is a specialized component of the CT computer system. It is capable of performing the massive calculations required for CT image reconstruction. (Wolbarst, 1993, p.302)
126. (b) Retrospective reconstruction uses scan or "raw" data to change the matrix, DFOV, center, and algorithm used for a CT image. The

slice thickness and SFOV are specifically used for data acquisition and cannot be altered retrospectively. (Berland, 1987, p.83)

127. (d) A decrease in matrix size causes a subsequent increase in pixel dimension. This larger size causes an increase in the number of x-rays passing through each pixel, thereby increasing the signal-to-noise ratio. (Wolbarst, 1993, p.331)
128. (d) The spatial resolution along the z axis is decreased when the pitch is increased. An increase in pitch causes less information to be acquired for each section reconstructed. This increase in pitch broadens the section sensitivity profile and reduces the spatial resolution. (Fishman et al., 1995, p.4)
129. (b) Prepatient collimation controls the slice thickness by reducing the size of the primary beam. This is accomplished with the use of lead shutters, which absorb the outer margins of the primary beam. Increases in prepatient collimation reduce patient dose by reducing the number of x-ray photons reaching the patient. (Seeram, 1994, p.98)
130. (c) The SFOV size is determined by the number of detectors activated during data acquisition. (Berland, 1987, p.45)
131. (b) Noise degrades the CT image with a grainy, mottled appearance. The terms quantum mottle and noise are often used interchangeably. (Curry et al., 1990, p.310)
132. (c) Noise or quantum mottle may be caused by absorption of an insufficient number of x-ray photons by the detectors. In this example, the technique chosen by the operator was most likely too low. (Curry et al., 1990, p.310)
133. (c) An average range of CT numbers for blood is +42 to +58. The CT number of any material is based on many factors, including the beam quality of a particular scanner. (Wolbarst, 1993, p.321)
134. (a) Owing to its high atomic number and relative stability, xenon gas is used in gas ionization CT detectors. (Seeram, 1994, p.101)
135. (b) The artifact shown in the figure most likely represents an out-of-field artifact. This relatively large patient was incorrectly positioned, and a portion of the anatomy lies outside of the scan field of view. This improperly centered anatomy interferes with the reference detectors, thus causing a streak artifact near the unscanned area. (Berland, 1987, p.155)
136. (d) The out-of-field artifact present in this image could be easily reduced by properly centering the patient within the SFOV. (Berland, 1987, p.155)
137. (d) The terms algorithm, kernel, and mathematical filter function may all be used interchangeably to describe the mathematical process used for the complex calculations required during CT image reconstruction. (Berland, 1987, p.79)

138. (a) It is important for the calibration of a CT scanner to be checked daily by the operator. CT units should be calibrated with their reference CT number for water at approximately zero Hounsfield units. The CT number for air should be at approximately −1000 Hounsfield units. (Seeram, 1994, p.235)
139. (d) The quality of multiplanar reformats can be greatly improved with the use of narrow, overlapping sections. (Seeram, 1994, p.172)
140. (c) The dense objects located in the abdomen of this patient most likely represent metallic surgical staples, which often appear in the postsurgical patient. (Berland, 1987, p.156)
141. (a) The azimuth setting is determined by the relationship between the x-ray tube and detectors during scout or localizer production. At a 0° azimuth, the x-ray tube and detectors do not rotate and remain above and below the patient, providing a frontal projection. (Seeram, 1994, p.175)
142. (c) Materials whose attenuation coefficients are less than that of water are assigned negative CT numbers. The CT number of a material is calculated by comparing the attenuation coefficient of the material with the attenuation coefficient of water. (Wolbarst, 1993, p.321)
143. (d) The window chosen for image display should always be tailored to the needs of the individual anatomy. The level should be set at an average value for the tissue of interest, with a width wide enough to include all variations within the region of interest. (Berland, 1987, p.127)
144. (c) Interpolation is a mathematical technique used in spiral CT. In interpolation, approximations of information above and below a section level are made to overcome the fact that a complete revolution of tube and detectors was not performed for each image. (Fishman et al., 1995, p.5)
145. (d) Predetector and postpatient collimation are synonymous. Both terms describe a device designed to remove scatter radiation before it reaches the detector. (Seeram, 1994, p.98)
146. (c) A voxel may be defined as a volume element. It is represented within a matrix by a pixel. (Seeram, 1994, p.63)
147. (b) The presence of metal within the patient causes a streak artifact on the image. This occurs as the dense metal absorbs a large amount of the radiation, interfering with the signal produced. (Seeram, 1994, p.213)
148. (c) Metallic dental fillings often cause a streak artifact during CT examinations of the head. (Chiu et al., 1995, p.37)
149. (b) The spatial resolution of a CT examination can be improved with the use of small focal spots, narrow sections, and large matrices. (Seeram, 1994, p.202)
150. (a) The term ray is used to describe the portion of the x-ray beam that falls on a single detector. (Seeram, 1994, p.87)

CHAPTER 6

Answer Key for Simulated Exam Two

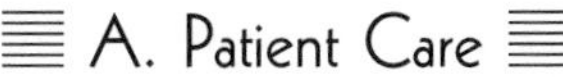

A. Patient Care

1. (b) The normal range for creatinine level is 0.6–1.5 mg/dL. The normal range for blood urea nitrogen (BUN) level is 8–23 mg/dL. Creatinine and BUN are laboratory values that may be used to evaluate the renal function of a patient scheduled to undergo a CT examination that includes iodinated intravenous contrast. (*The Merck Manual*, 1987, p.2412)
2. (d) Informed consent must be obtained from the patient before any invasive procedure is undertaken. The components of informed consent include a thorough explanation of the examination, any possible risks as well as proposed benefits, and alternative examinations. (Adler and Carlton, 1994, p.350)
3. (c) Ionic contrast materials are salts that separate into independent charged particles when placed in aqueous solutions. The charged particles are typically termed anions and cations. (Katzberg, 1992, p.3)
4. (b) A butterfly needle should be inserted at an angle of 15° for the intravenous administration of contrast material. The vein should be properly stabilized and the needle inserted gently with the bevel facing upward. (Adler and Carlton, 1994, p.294)
5. (a) The course of an infection can be divided into four stages. The incubation stage begins when a pathogenic organism enters the host. The prodromal stage is characterized by the appearance of early signs and symptoms of the disease process. The active or full stage includes the maximal appearance of the signs and symptoms of the disease. During the last stage, convalescence, the symptoms begin to decrease and may eventually completely subside. (Torres, 1993, p.29)

6. (d) The normal range for systolic blood pressure in adults is 95–140 mm Hg. Systolic pressure is the measurement of blood pressure at its peak during contraction of the heart. (Adler and Carlton, 1994, p.181)
7. (c) To reduce the possibility of headaches, the patient should rest for 8–24 hours with the head slightly elevated (35°–45°) after a CT examination involving an intrathecal injection of contrast material. (Torres, 1993, p.241)
8. (c) Urticaria is a common adverse reaction to iodinated intravenous contrast material. It is characterized by the presence of wheals or localized skin eruptions. It is commonly referred to as hives. (Copstead, 1995, p.1067)
9. (a) The fetus is most susceptible to the harmful effects of ionizing radiation during the first trimester of the gestation period. (Adler and Carlton, 1994, p.43)
10. (c) The American Hospital Association drafted *A Patient's Bill of Rights* in 1973. Included among the 12 "rights" are the patient's right to considerate and respectful care and the right to refuse treatment. Release of the patient's diagnostic examination is not an inherent right and is at the discretion of the physicians involved. (Torres, 1993, p.6)
11. (a) Patients suffering from vagal reactions to iodinated contrast material show symptoms of hypotension and bradycardia. Treatment includes increasing blood pressure with intravenous fluids and intravenous administration of atropine to block vagal stimulation of the heart. (Katzberg, 1992, p.25)
12. (d) The correct order for the scheduling of these procedures is the CT study first, followed by the barium enema, and the gastrointestinal series last. Dense barium causes a streak artifact on the CT image, so it is important for CT to be performed first. The barium administered during a gastrointestinal series could interfere with interpretation of a diagnostic enema study. (Adler and Carlton, 1994, p.320)
13. (b) The viscosity of a fluid is a measure of the ability of the fluid to flow. A fluid with a high viscosity is relatively thick and flows slowly. The viscosity of a solution may vary with changes in temperature. (Katzberg, 1992, p.6)
14. (c) The normal range of respirations for a child is 20–30 breaths per minute. (Adler and Carlton, 1994, p.181)
15. (d) The intravenous method of drug administration allows for direct entry of the drug into the bloodstream. This results in the immediate effect of the drug on a patient. (Torres, 1993, p.217)
16. (a) When performing cardiopulmonary resuscitation, the first action is always to secure an open airway. Mouth-to-mouth or any other type of oxygen support is then initiated. The third action is external cardiac

compression after a lack of pulse has been determined. (Torres, 1993, p.98)

17. (b) Before the intravenous injection of contrast media, a tourniquet is placed proximal to the injection site. The tourniquet helps to distend the vein, making needle insertion easier. (Adler and Carlton, 1994, p.294)
18. (d) The high atomic number of iodine causes it to attenuate a large portion of the primary beam. Introducing iodine into tissue changes the subject contrast of the enhanced anatomic area. (Tortorici and Apfel, 1995, p.19)
19. (a) Severe reactions to iodinated contrast material include anaphylaxis, shock, cardiac arrest, and death. Urticaria and vomiting may be considered mild or moderate reactions, depending on their severity. (Putman and Ravin, 1994, p.1068)
20. (c) Antiseptic solution is often applied to the patient's skin before an invasive procedure such as a CT-guided needle biopsy is performed. The antiseptic should be applied in a circular motion, beginning at the center and working outward. This ensures that the center location for the procedure has been thoroughly cleansed. (Torres, 1993, p.179)
21. (b) The Compton reaction is responsible for the production of scatter radiation. In the Compton reaction, an x-ray photon strikes an outer shell orbital electron of an atom of tissue. The orbital electron is ejected and is termed a recoil electron. The incident x-ray photon retains a part of its original energy and continues on in a different direction as a scattered photon. Because the CT technologist is never exposed to primary radiation, Compton scatter is the major source of occupational exposure. (Curry et al., 1994, p.65)
22. (d) Proper communication with the patient before the start of any CT examination is extremely important. A thorough explanation of the procedure with a detailed set of instructions helps to reduce patient anxiety and improve cooperation in obtaining a high-quality study. (Adler and Carlton, 1994, p.120)
23. (c) The osmolality of a contrast material is a measure of the number of particles per kilogram of water. Osmolality is a factor in determining the potential for adverse reaction from iodinated contrast material. Ionic contrast media, which dissolve into a large number of anions and cations in solution, have an average osmolality between 1000 and 2400 mOsm/kg. (Tortorici and Apfel, 1995, p.21)
24. (d) The purpose of a biphasic contrast injection is to complete scanning of the liver before the onset of equilibrium, when hepatic lesions could be obscured. A biphasic injection consists of a rapid initial flow rate followed by a slower rate of injection. (Fishman et al., 1995, p.13)
25. (b) Fomites are objects that have been contaminated by an infectious organism or microbe. The spread of the infection may occur when a

person comes into contact with the fomite. This is an indirect means of infection transmission. (Torres, 1993, p.29)

26. (c) The term for difficulty in swallowing is dysphagia. The prefix *dys* denotes difficulty or painful, and the suffix *phagia* means to eat or swallow. (*Mosby's Medical Dictionary*, 1994)
27. (c) Platelets are a component of blood that are responsible for coagulation. The normal range for platelet count is 150,000–400,000/mm^3 of blood. A patient's platelet count becomes important when performing an invasive CT procedure. The platelet count of the patient must be within the normal range to ensure that abnormal bleeding does not occur. (*Mosby's Medical Dictionary,* 1994)
28. (b) Angiocatheters are most often used for contrast administration with an automatic injector. The stability of an angiocatheter stands up well to the high pressure of an automatic injector. Infuse-A-Ports and port-A-Caths are usually not used for contrast administration. (Katzberg, 1992, p.75)
29. (a) A stochastic effect of radiation exposure is one having no threshold dose. Common examples of stochastic radiation effects are genetic mutations and cancer. (Curry et al., 1994, p.377)
30. (c) Patients may be placed in a higher risk group for an adverse reaction to iodinated contrast based on several factors, including their previous allergic history and physical condition. Patients considered to be at high risk for adverse reaction should be administered nonionic contrast material. (Katzberg, 1992, p.71)

B. Imaging Procedures

31. (d) The abdominal aorta descends to the level of the fourth lumbar vertebra, where it bifurcates into the left and right common iliac arteries. (Clemente, 1985, p.731)
32. (b) Quantitative CT is used to measure the mineral content of bone. Density measurements of the patient's bone are compared with density measurements of a reference phantom. The bone mineral density values are compared with normal values to assess osteoporosis. (Seeram, 1994, p.175)
33. (c) Soft-tissue or standard algorithm selection is made when imaging soft-tissue structures such as those found in the mediastinum. (Seeram, 1994, p.271)
34. (d) Left pulmonary artery (Bo et al., 1990, p.86)
35. (c) Number 5 corresponds to the right primary bronchus. (Bo et al., 1990, p.86)
36. (a) Descending aorta (Bo et al., 1990, p.86)
37. (b) The density of the mass indicates that it consists of fatty tissue. A lipoma is a benign mass consisting of fat cells. An angiomyolipoma is a common benign mass found in the kidney and it consists of muscle

cells, blood vessels, and fat. The average CT value range for fat is −50 to −100 Hounsfield units. (Moss et al., 1992, p.971)

38. (d) Pneumothorax is one of the most common complications from CT-guided needle biopsy of the lung. The term pneumothorax describes a collection of air in the pleural space. A pneumothorax causes a portion of the lung to collapse, often requiring placement of a chest tube to reinflate the lung. (Moss et al., 1992, p.332)
39. (b) Semicircular canal (Chiu et al., 1995, p.58)
40. (c) Petrous bone (Chiu et al., 1995, p.28)
41. (d) An extremely wide window should be used to display images containing tissues with varying density ranges. A width such as 4000 is sufficient to display the dense bone of the mastoid tip and internal auditory canals. The level is set at the approximate average value of the tissues displayed. A level of +250 is the approximate average of all tissues within this anatomic region. (Berland, 1987, p.123)
42. (b) Sphenoid sinus (Chiu et al., 1995, p.65)
43. (b) The SFOV chosen for any CT study must be larger than the anatomic part of interest. Specific SFOV choices, such as that for the head, incorporate special correction factors for their respective anatomic areas and should be used when applicable. (Seeram, 1994, p.271)
44. (c) Suspended respiration at the end of full expiration is the most reproducible point in the respiratory cycle. This results in less misregistration artifact during CT examinations of the abdomen (Chiu et al., 1995, p.112)
45. (c) During CT examination of the pelvis, both intravenous and oral contrast material are commonly administered. Intravenous contrast is important in differentiating pelvic blood vessels from lymph nodes. Oral contrast opacifies the small and large colon and greatly improves their visualization. Oil-based contrast media are not commonly used for CT procedures. (Katzberg, 1992, p.78)
46. (b) Number 3 corresponds to the common carotid artery. (Bo et al., 1990, p.46)
47. (a) Internal jugular vein (Bo et al., 1990, p.46)
48. (c) Sternocleidomastoid muscle (Bo et al., 1990, p.44)
49. (c) A common range of contrast volume for an intrathecal injection during post-myelographic CT is 12–14 mL in an adult patient. The total volume should not exceed approximately 17 mL, keeping the dose below 3 g of iodine. (Katzberg, 1992, p.114)
50. (d) The localizer or scout image for a CT study of the abdomen should include from above the diaphragm to the level of the iliac crest. Routine studies of the abdomen require axial sections including the liver in its entirety to the beginning of the pelvis at the iliac crest. (Berland, 1987, p.228)

51. (a) Lateral condyle (Bo et al., 1990, p.303)
52. (d) Intercondylar fossa (Clemente, 1985, p.280)
53. (c) During CT examinations of the knee, patients are commonly positioned in the supine position. In the figure, the patella is positioned superiorly, indicating the supine position. If the patient had been in the prone position, the image would have to be rotated on the screen 180° to be placed in the proper orientation. (Seeram, 1994, p.299)
54. (b) Glucagon may be used to reduce peristaltic motion contractions during CT imaging of the abdomen and pelvis. A 1-mg intravenous injection just before scanning is a typical dose. (Moss et al., 1992, p.1183)
55. (c) Benign prostatic hypertrophy is a nonmalignant enlargement of the prostate commonly seen in men older than 50 years of age. (*The Merck Manual*, 1987, p.1635)
56. (b) Left subclavian artery (Bo et al., 1990, p.78)
57. (a) Right brachiocephalic vein (Bo et al., 1990, p.78)
58. (c) Left brachiocephalic vein (Bo et al., 1990, p.78)
59. (c) Number 4 corresponds to the left common carotid artery. (Bo et al., 1990, p.78)
60. (c) The diagnosis of hemangioma is confirmed on CT by evaluation of its pattern of enhancement. Hemangiomas enhance from the periphery inward until they become isodense with the surrounding hepatic tissue. Once isodense, the hemangioma attenuates the beam the same as the hepatic tissue. The CT numbers of the hemangioma and hepatic tissue become equal and they may become impossible to differentiate. (Moss et al., 1992, p.764)
61. (b) Spiral or helical CT offers many advantages over conventional CT. Complete anatomic areas are scanned in very short times owing to continuous acquisition of data and no interscan delay. Because no delays are needed, entire volumes of information may be obtained, often during only one breath hold. This reduces misregistration artifacts associated with inconsistent patient breathing. There is no reduction in patient dose with the use of spiral CT. (Seeram, 1994, p.114)
62. (b) Stomach (Bo et al., 1990, p.136)
63. (d) The location of the liver on the inferior portion of the image indicates that this patient is in the right lateral decubitus position. (Gedgaudas-McClees and Torres, 1990, p.139)
64. (b) The right lateral decubitus position is often used to differentiate the pancreatic head and the duodenum. (Putman and Ravin, 1994, p.990)
65. (a) Right ureter (Bo et al., 1990, p.136)
66. (c) The choroid plexus and pineal gland are common areas of calcification in the brain. These areas of increased attenuation and density are easily identified on the CT image. (Putman and Ravin, 1994, p.131)

67. (a) Barium sulfate is normally too dense to be useful in CT imaging. Even when barium is diluted with water, its high attenuation characteristics can cause streaking artifacts on the CT image. Some commercially available CT oral contrast media preparations do contain barium sulfate in 1%–3% suspensions. The suspension contains additives that prevent settling of the barium sulfate, which could cause inhomogeneous opacification of the gastrointestinal system. (Katzberg, 1992, p.203)
68. (c) Lamina (Clemente, 1985, p.131)
69. (c) Body (Bo et al., 1990, p.44)
70. (c) Number 1 corresponds to the foramen transversarium. (Clemente, 1985, p.131)
71. (d) The diagnosis of a simple cyst is accurately made with the proper CT examination. Precontrast and postcontrast images must be obtained to measure enhancement. The attenuation values for the cystic area should be at or near zero. The diagnoses of appendicitis, a renal stone, and diverticulitis can be made without the intravenous injection of contrast material. (Gedgaudas-McClees and Torres, 1990, p.144)
72. (a) Routine CT scanning of the head should be performed with the gantry angled 15° above the orbitomeatal line. This produces axial sections of the brain while limiting beam hardening artifacts and direct orbital exposure. (Chiu et al., 1995, p.21)
73. (c) Ultrafast CT scanners are designed to acquire information at an extremely rapid rate. With the use of electron beam technology, ultrafast CT scanners can greatly reduce cardiac and pulmonary motion, allowing detailed evaluation of anatomic areas such as the coronary arteries. (Seeram, 1994, p.184)
74. (b) The air–fluid level present in the bladder indicates that the patient was administered intravenous contrast material. The rectum is not opacified, thus giving no indication of oral or enema administration of contrast material. (Berland, 1987, p.239)
75. (a) Seminal vesicles (Bo et al., 1990, p.202)
76. (d) Femoral artery (Bo et al., 1990, p.202)
77. (b) Sartorius muscle (Bo et al., 1990, p.202)
78. (d) High-resolution CT (HRCT) of the chest is used to examine diffuse pulmonary disease. This technique offers excellent visualization of the lungs, airways, and pulmonary hilum. HRCT involves the use of narrow sections (1–3 mm) and a high-resolution algorithm. (Seeram, 1994, p.296)
79. (c) Dynamic scanning is a common technique used during imaging of the chest and abdomen. It involves the bolus administration of contrast material, immediately followed by rapid scanning through the area of interest. The interscan delays are limited to the minimum

amount allowed by the tube cooling requirements of the scanner. (Berland, 1987, p.206)

80. (b) Subdural hematomas are collections of blood that occur throughout the subdural space after traumatic injury to the head. An acute subdural hematoma is one that clinically manifests during the first 24 hours after the injury. During this stage, the hematoma appears hyperdense when compared with normal brain tissue owing to the initial clotting that has occurred and the concentration of hemoglobin in fresh blood. (Putman and Ravin, 1994, p.188)
81. (b) Anterior superior iliac spine (Wicke, 1994, p.46)
82. (c) The patient was positioned in the dorsal recumbent (supine) position with arms placed overhead. This is the standard position for localizer production during CT studies of the chest, abdomen, and pelvis. (Seeram, 1994, p.296)
83. (c) Splenic flexure (Wicke, 1994, p.127)
84. (c) The localizer (scout) image shown includes the areas of the abdomen and pelvis. The chest is not included in its entirety, and therefore, this scout could not be used to prescribe a CT study of the chest. CT studies of the abdomen only should be programmed from a scout including the area from above the diaphragm to the level of the iliac crests. This eliminates unnecessary exposure to the pelvis. (Berland, 1987, p.228)
85. (d) Obturator foramen (Wicke, 1994, p.127)
86. (d) During a CT examination of the lumbar spine, a foam cushion should be placed under the patient's flexed knees. This reduces strain on the lower back, making the patient more comfortable and cooperative. It also reduces the lordotic curve of the lumbar spine, allowing for more accurate imaging of the intervertebral disk spaces. (Chiu et al., 1995, p.161)
87. (c) Numerous factors may be regarded as contraindications to iodinated contrast material administration. They include prior severe reaction to contrast, renal failure, pheochromocytoma, acute sickle cell anemia, and multiple myeloma. An allergic history to shellfish is not always a definite contraindication to iodinated contrast material. Depending on the severity of the allergic history, non-ionic contrast may be used or the patient may be premedicated with corticosteroids, antihistamines, or both. (Katzberg, 1992, p.70)
88. (d) Pulmonary nodules appearing on CT examinations of the lungs may be determined as benign if their average density is more than +164 Hounsfield units. Although studies have yielded conflicting results in this area, researchers tend to agree that density values approaching +200 Hounsfield units make the benign diagnosis more certain. (Moss et al., 1992, p.176)
89. (d) Humeral head (Bo et al., 1990, p.326)

90. (b) Glenoid fossa (Bo et al., 1990, p.326)
91. (a) Multiplanar reconstruction studies are best performed using narrow sections acquired with no spacing or, preferably, an overlap. The 3- × 3-mm selection would provide the greatest detail among the given choices. (Seeram, 1994, p.252)
92. (c) The posterior horn of the lateral ventricle contains cerebrospinal fluid and does not enhance after the administration of intravenous contrast material. Areas having a good blood supply, such as the cranial blood vessels, choroid plexus, and dura mater, enhance during a contrast study of the brain. (Seeram, 1994, p.271)
93. (a) Insertion of a tampon during the CT examination of the pelvis dilates the vagina and fills it with negative contrast (air). This makes for easier visualization of the vagina and its relationship with surrounding structures. (Chiu et al., 1995, p.117)
94. (c) Pancreas (Bo et al., 1990, p.136)
95. (d) For a CT examination of the abdomen, oral contrast should be administered in volumes of approximately 500 mL, 15–30 minutes before the examination. An additional 300 mL should be given just before the study. This method of administration should provide adequate opacification of the stomach and small bowel. (Berland, 1987, p.231)
96. (b) Adrenal gland (Bo et al., 1990, p.128)
97. (b) Number 1 corresponds to the left lobe of the liver. (Bo et al., 1990, p. 130)
98. (c) The sagittal plane divides the body into right and left portions. The coronal plane divides the body into anterior and posterior portions. The axial (transverse, horizontal) plane occurs at right angles to the sagittal and coronal planes and divides the body into superior and inferior portions. (Clemente, 1985, p.2)
99. (c) Intravenous contrast administration during a CT examination of the pelvis is valuable for several reasons. The bladder is easily visualized when filled with contrast, and differentiation between blood vessels and enlarged pelvic lymph nodes is improved. The rectosigmoid junction may be better visualized once opacification has been attained through the use of oral or enema contrast administration. (Katzberg, 1992, p.79; Berland and Lincoln, 1987, p.239)
100. (d) Genu of corpus callosum (Bo et al., 1990, p.12)
101. (b) Falx cerebri (Bo et al., 1990, p.12)
102. (b) Number 2 corresponds to the internal capsule. (Bo et al., 1990, p.12)
103. (a) Pineal gland (Bo et al., 1990, p.12)
104. (a) During a CT examination of the spine, the DFOV should be one that displays the spine enlarged on the monitor. Commonly referred to as targeting, this technique provides the viewer with an enlarged

image of the spine without the loss of detail that accompanies magnification of the CT image. Although in this example the patient measures 40 cm across, the DFOV of 15 cm is sufficient to target the spine and enlarge its image on the viewing monitor. (Seeram, 1994, p.271)

105. (d) Diverticulosis is the presence of small pouch-like openings in the wall of the colon. The term diverticulitis is used when the diverticula become inflamed. (Copstead, 1995, p.733)

C. Physics and Instrumentation

106. (d) The Lambert-Beer law is properly written as $I = I_0e^{-\mu x}$. This important exponential equation describes how x-ray photons are attenuated as they travel through matter and is used to calculate the linear attenuation coefficient (μ) of the tissue being imaged. (Seeram, 1994, p.70)
107. (c) A pixel is an element of the digital image. It is located in a matrix and is a two-dimensional representation of a voxel. When CT numbers are calculated for voxels (volume elements) of tissue, the pixel is assigned that number and a subsequent shade of gray. The pixel may be defined as a picture (*pix*) element (*el*), or the smallest component of the digital image. (Chiu et al., 1995, p.6)
108. (b) Interpolation is a mathematical technique used in the reconstruction process of the spiral CT image. It involves the estimation of an unknown value from information above and below it. (Seeram, 1994, p.114)
109. (b) When calculated by a formula comparing the attenuation coefficient of tissue with that of water, materials whose coefficient is greater than that of water are assigned positive CT numbers. (Wolbarst, 1993, p.321)
110. (a) CT demonstrates improved low-contrast resolution when compared with conventional radiography. The CT system is extremely sensitive to small changes in tissue density, and it removes the problem of superimposition, both of which lead to greater low-contrast resolution. (Seeram, 1994, p.69)
111. (a) The Austrian mathematician Radon was responsible for some of the earliest scientific research for the reconstruction principles used in CT. In 1917, he proved that it was possible to build an image of an object using an extremely large set of its projections. (Seeram, 1994, p.2)
112. (b) The silver halide crystal is not used as detector material in CT. (Seeram, 1994, p.101)
113. (d) Water has a CT number at or near zero. This area most likely represents a hepatic cyst. (Seeram, 1994, p.74)
114. (c) Water has an average attenuation coefficient value of 0.206. (Seeram, 1994, p.75)

115. (b) The width of a window used to display a CT image of the abdomen should be within the range of 350–600 Hounsfield units. This range allows for excellent visualization of the soft-tissue structures. (Berland, 1987, p.127)
116. (c) Owing to the high-energy beam used in CT, the Compton interaction is the predominant interaction between x-ray and matter. CT scanners use between 120 and 140 kVp, yielding x-ray energies with averages of 70–80 keV. (Wolbarst, 1993, p.321)
117. (d) The contrast of a CT image is controlled by the spatial frequencies of the tissues within the section. Tissues of differing densities are represented electronically by different spatial frequencies. Adjacent tissues with similar densities or areas of tissue with minimal differences in density are represented by low spatial frequencies. (Berland, 1987, p.33)
118. (c) Ring artifacts are associated with the use of third-generation CT scanners. Both the x-ray tube and the detector array rotate about the patient with third-generation scanners. A malfunctioning detector or series of detectors in a third-generation CT scanner will cause a ring artifact to appear on the image owing to the rotational nature of the detector array. (Seeram, 1994, p.215)
119. (c) A byte is a series of 8 bits. Bits and bytes are part of the binary language used by computers to process information. (Wolbarst, 1993, p.299)
120. (d) The limiting resolution of a modern CT scanner is approximately 20 lp/cm (lp = line pair). This varies greatly with scan factors and is considerably less than that of projection radiography. (Seeram, 1994, p.202)
121. (a) Thorough communication between the technologist and the patient is vital in ensuring superior examination quality. If the patient has been informed of the examination process, anxiety may be reduced and cooperation is improved. During all CT procedures, the patient must be instructed to be still to reduce motion artifact on the CT images. (Chiu et al., 1995, p.11)
122. (c) The radiographic film used to archive CT images is a single-emulsion film that may be used with multiformat or laser cameras. Light is used to expose the film within the multiformat camera, whereas a laser beam exposes the film in a laser camera. (Berland, 1987, p.131)
123. (d) The filtered back-projection or convolution method of image reconstruction is used by most modern CT scanners. (Moss et al., 1992, p.1357)
124. (c) Fourth-generation CT scanners operate with a rotating x-ray tube and a stationary ring of detectors. Some fourth-generation scanners also use a rotating x-ray tube with a nutating detector ring. (Seeram, 1994, p.89)

125. (b) Noise appears on the CT image as an inaccuracy in CT number. The noise of a CT scanner may be measured by scanning a homogeneous object such as a water phantom. Fluctuations in CT number from pixel to pixel indicate the presence of noise. (Seeram, 1994, p.209)
126. (c) Beam hardening occurs as the x-ray beam traverses the patient. The x-ray beam used in CT is composed of x-ray photons with numerous different energy levels. The heterogeneous beam undergoes an increase in average photon energy as it passes through the patient and the lower energy photons are absorbed. (Seeram, 1994, p.214)
127. (c) When the cathode of an x-ray tube is heated, electrons are released through the process of thermionic emission. It is these electrons that are then accelerated toward the anode for x-ray production. (Curry et al., 1994, p.11)
128. (d) The signal-to-noise ratio of a CT image is increased when a larger amount of x-ray photons are absorbed by the detectors. Only an increase in aperture size (section width) would accomplish that from the given choices. (Wolbarst, 1993, p.331)
129. (b) A straight line artifact on a scanogram (pilot) image is most likely caused by a malfunctioning detector in both third- and fourth-generation scanners. As the patient travels through the gantry, the faulty detector does not record any information, leading to the appearance of a blank line on the image. (Berland, 1987, p.148)
130. (c) The CT dose index (CTDI) is used to quantify the radiation dose received by the patient during a CT scan. It involves the use of an ionization chamber to accurately measure radiation exposure for a given set of technical factors. (Seeram, 1994, p.221)
131. (b) The DFOV may be calculated by multiplying the pixel dimension by the matrix size. In this example, one side of the pixel measures 0.75 mm and the matrix used is 320^2. The DFOV is 240 mm or 24 cm. (Seeram, 1994, p.79)
132. (a) The spatial resolution of a CT scanner can be measured by studying the amount of blurring that occurs around a point within the CT image. Known as the point spread function, this image unsharpness may be graphically represented. The spatial resolution can then be quantified by measuring the graph at half its maximum value. This measurement is called the full width at half-maximum and is used to illustrate the spatial resolution of a CT scanner. (Seeram, 1994, p.198)
133. (b) The average photon energy of the primary beam used in CT is approximately 70 keV. The average photon energy of any radiographic primary beam is approximately 30%–40% of the applied kilovoltage. The average photon energy of the CT beam is increased slightly through beam filtration. (Curry et al., 1994, p.319)
134. (c) The edge gradient effect occurs when the CT x-ray beam passes through areas of abrupt changes in density, which are represented by

high spatial frequencies. This type of streak artifact commonly occurs at the interface of dense bone and soft tissue in anatomic areas such as the brain. (Berland, 1987, p.149)

135. (b) Streak artifacts due to the heterogeneous nature of the CT x-ray beam may be reduced with increases in the average photon energy of the beam. Increases in kVp and filtration would accomplish this. This type of artifact may also be reduced with a decrease in aperture size, which helps to minimize the edge gradient effect. (Berland, 1987, p.150)
136. (c) The level chosen for a given window setting should correspond to the average density value of the tissues of interest. Areas of soft tissue, such as the brain, are often displayed at window levels of approximately +50 Hounsfield units. (Seeram, 1994, p.170)
137. (a) Modern CT scanners use large matrices for image reconstruction and display. Typical sizes include 320^2, 512^2, and 1024^2. (Moss et al., 1992, p.1359)
138. (c) Collimation occurs as lead shutters close down upon the beam, limiting its projected area. Constructed of lead, the collimator shutters absorb portions of the primary beam, thereby reducing its intensity. (Bushberg et al., 1994, p.262)
139. (d) Statistical noise is a term that may be used for quantum noise or mottle. Caused by an insufficient number of photons being detected, this type of noise appears as a graininess on the CT image. (Seeram, 1994, p.209)
140. (c) The reduced low-contrast resolution of the scanner is most likely caused by increased noise. When the noise level of a CT image increases, the low-contrast resolution decreases. Decreased patient dose implies that the signal-to-noise ratio has decreased, thus increasing the noise level of the image. The same situation applies for an increase in electronic noise. (Seeram, 1994, p.238)
141. (a) The high-frequency generator used to produce the three-phase power used in modern CT scanners is located inside the gantry. It may be positioned in a corner of the gantry or fixed to the rotating tube assembly. (Seeram, 1994, p.96)
142. (c) The threshold setting is used to include and exclude information during the three-dimensional reconstruction of a CT scan. For example, a high threshold (+150 Hounsfield units) may be set to produce a three-dimensional model of a bony structure. This threshold eliminates any density value less than +150 Hounsfield units from the data set. The reconstructed three-dimensional model would include only bone tissue, or any other substance with a Hounsfield value of more than +150. (Seeram, 1994, p.254)
143. (d) Each component of CT image quality may be affected—either positively or negatively—by the CT technologist. Spatial resolution is

affected by geometric factors such as focal spot size and slice thickness. Contrast resolution may be altered by slice thickness, algorithm selection, and noise. The noise level of an image depends on several factors, including patient dose and pixel dimension. Each of these factors must be considered by the CT technologist to provide high-quality CT studies. (Seeram, 1994, p.200)

144. (d) The x-ray tube and data acquisition system are housed within the gantry of a CT scanner. The gantry aperture is the circular opening through which the patient moves during scanning. (Seeram, 1994, p.143)
145. (c) Partial volume artifact can be reduced in several ways. With conventional CT, the area is rescanned with a narrower section thickness. This reduces the partial volume artifact but increases patient dose. Spiral CT allows for retrospective reconstruction at any location along the acquired volume. This may be helpful in positioning the area of interest within the voxel length for improved accuracy. Because slice thickness is controlled by the collimation of the x-ray beam, it cannot be adjusted retrospectively. (Berland, 1987, p.159)
146. (d) The matrix size indicates the number of pixels across and the number of pixels down. A 512 × 512 matrix has 262,144 pixels, which is calculated by squaring 512. (Wolbarst, 1993, p.320)
147. (b) The streaking artifact was most likely caused by surgical staples. This type of metallic streaking artifact is caused by the edge gradient effect. (Berland, 1987, p.156)
148. (c) The value of a pixel in Hounsfield units is calculated through a comparison of the linear attenuation coefficient (μ) of a voxel of tissue to that of water. (Seeram, 1994, p.74)
149. (d) Capable of storing between 200 and 3200 MB of digital information, the magnetic optical disk has the highest storage capacity of the archival media listed. (Seeram, 1994, p.35)
150. (b) The contrast resolution of a CT scanner refers to the ability of the system to differentiate objects with similar densities. This is also commonly referred to as low-contrast resolution or the sensitivity of the CT scanner. (Seeram, 1994, p.206)

CHAPTER 7

Answer Key for Simulated Exam Three

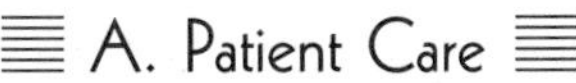

A. Patient Care

1. (c) A vagal reaction to iodinated intravenous contrast must be recognized early so that proper initial treatment is provided. A combination of bradycardia (heart rate less than 50 beats per minute) and hypotension (systolic pressure less than 80 mm Hg) indicates a vagal reaction. (Katzberg, 1992, p.24)
2. (b) Proper hand washing technique requires a minimum of 30 seconds. The technologist should use soap and warm water with a firm circular motion. (Torres, 1993, p.34)
3. (c) The purpose of a consent form is to educate the patient regarding all aspects of the procedure to be performed. A signed consent form indicates that the patient thoroughly understands the procedure. There are several components of a proper consent form, including a statement authorizing the health professional to perform the procedure; a full explanation of the procedure with the involved risks, benefits, and possible alternatives; a statement indicating that the patient understands the procedure; and the patient's signature. (Adler and Carlton, 1994, p.350)
4. (d) The partial thromboplastin time indicates the coagulation time of a patient's blood. It is often abbreviated as PTT. (*The Merck Manual*, 1987, p.1152)
5. (d) Non-ionic contrast material has a lower incidence of adverse reaction when compared with ionic contrast material. Non-ionic media are also higher in cost and offer no reduction in renal toxicity. (Adler and Carlton, 1994, p.314)
6. (a) Certain harmful effects of exposure to diagnostic x-ray beams, such as cancer formation and genetic mutations, are said to be stochas-

tic. A stochastic effect is one that has no threshold dose but increases in probability with increasing dose. Modern theories regarding the relationship of radiation exposure and biologic response are considered stochastic. (Curry et al., 1990, p.377)

7. (a) The gauge of a needle signifies its bore dimension or lumen size. The gauge of a needle increases as its lumen size decreases. Therefore, a 19-gauge needle has a larger lumen than a 23-gauge needle. (Adler and Carlton, 1994, p.287)
8. (c) The use of automatic injectors does not decrease the cost to the patient when compared with the manual bolus technique. Automatic injectors do offer decreased injection times, consistent administration, and increased enhancement. (Seeram, 1994, p.295)
9. (b) The maximum dose of intravenous iodinated contrast should not exceed 3 mg/kg body weight during pediatric CT examinations. Contrast loads in excess of this have been reported to cause acute osmolar poisoning in children. (Katzberg, 1992, p.208)
10. (c) The normal prothrombin time is approximately 10–12 seconds. This test is used to evaluate the coagulation ability of a patient scheduled to undergo an invasive CT procedure. (*The Merck Manual*, 1987, p.1154)
11. (c) Examples of moderate or intermediate reactions to iodinated intravenous contrast include severe vomiting, dyspnea, syncope (lightheadedness), chest pain, and seizures. Shock is an example of a severe reaction. (Putman and Ravin, 1994, p.1068)
12. (c) Patient dose varies widely among different CT examinations and scanners and is greatly affected by technical factor selection. An average range of patient skin dose during a CT study of the head is 2–4 cGy. One centigray (cGy) is equal to one rad. (Berland, 1987, p.40)
13. (d) During a one-person cardiopulmonary resuscitation attempt, 15 chest compressions should be done, followed by two ventilations. The person must be checked at regular intervals for the presence of respiration and pulse. (Adler and Carlton, 1994, p.264)
14. (b) The contrast bottle should remain at a distance of 18–24 inches above the patient during an intravenous drip infusion. Placing the bottle below the patient allows blood to return into the tubing. (Torres, 1993, p.223)
15. (a) The term emesis is commonly used in place of the term vomit. An emesis basin is one that is curved to fit against a patient's neck to collect vomitus. (*Mosby's Medical Dictionary*, 1994)
16. (b) Strict isolation precautions are used with patients at risk of infection owing to immunosuppression or some other form of debilitating disease. This type of precaution technique was previously referred to as protective or reverse isolation. (Torres, 1993, p.39)

17. (c) Intrathecal injections of iodinated contrast material are commonly used in the CT evaluation of the lumbar spine. This type of injection introduces contrast directly into the subarachnoid space. (Chiu et al., 1995, p.162)
18. (a) Severe reactions to intravenous iodinated contrast media occur in less than 1% of all patients. Examples of severe reactions include shock, myocardial infarction, and death. (Katzberg, 1992, p.166)
19. (d) Solu-Cortef is a brand name for hydrocortisone, which is a type of corticosteroid. Solu-Cortef, or other types of corticosteroids, may be used during the treatment of anaphylactoid reactions to iodinated contrast materials. (Katzberg, 1992, p.24)
20. (c) The total injection time may be calculated by dividing the contrast volume by the flow rate. In this example, the flow rate is 1.5 mL/sec for a total of 150 mL. The time required for this injection would be 100 seconds. (Snopek, 1992, p.49)
21. (b) Serum creatinine levels are the most accurate and dependable laboratory measure of renal function. The blood urea nitrogen (BUN) level may be affected by many variables and is not suited as a test for renal function by itself. BUN levels are usually evaluated in conjunction with creatinine levels for a more accurate measurement of renal function. (*The Merck Manual*, 1987, p.1561)
22. (b) The normal range for diastolic blood pressure in adults is 60–90 mm Hg. Diastolic pressure is the measurement of blood pressure at its lowest point, in between contractions of the heart. (Adler and Carlton, 1994, p.181)
23. (c) Prior reactions to contrast media and a history of asthma are factors that increase the incidence of adverse reaction to iodinated contrast media. It is therefore vital to question the patient regarding these factors before contrast administration. Infection with human immunodeficiency virus and hepatitis virus does not increase the incidence of adverse reaction to iodinated contrast media. Because universal precautions govern protection of all patients and health care professionals, it is of no use to question the patient regarding these factors. (Katzberg, 1992, p.70; Adler and Carlton, 1994, p.209)
24. (d) The escape of contrast material from a needle or blood vessel into the subcutaneous tissues is called extravasation. It is also sometimes referred to as infiltration. (*Mosby's Medical Dictionary*, 1994)
25. (a) Each hospital or private outpatient facility has its own specific protocols regarding patient preparation for CT examinations. However, when possible, patients should refrain from eating for some time before their examination. Avoiding eating before a CT scan of the abdomen and pelvis reduces nausea and vomiting from contrast injections, decreases patient discomfort from bladder filling during the study, and ensures gastric emptying for more accurate diagnoses. An

empty stomach also makes it easier for the patient to consume the necessary oral contrast. (Berland, 1987, p.199)

26. (b) Barium sulfate is not water soluble and is not easily absorbed by the body. If it leaks out of the digestive tract owing to perforation, it may cause peritonitis. (Katzberg, 1992, p.199)
27. (c) The pitch of a spiral CT scan is the ratio of the table speed to the section thickness. When the pitch is increased, a volume of anatomy is scanned with a reduced number of tube and detector rotations. This allows for reduced patient dose while the necessary anatomic area is scanned. (Fishman and Brooke, 1995, p.4)
28. (d) Administration of an antihistamine is the usual treatment for the development of urticaria (hives) after the injection of iodinated contrast. (Katzberg, 1992, p.23)
29. (b) The term dyspnea may be defined as the condition of difficult breathing. (*Mosby's Medical Dictionary*, 1994)
30. (a) Medical asepsis is the reduction in number of infectious agents without the complete elimination of the organisms. It is accomplished through the use of soap, water, and many other types of disinfectant materials. (Adler and Carlton, 1994, p.207)

B. Imaging Procedures

31. (b) Wilms' tumor is a specific type of renal mass that develops from immature renal parenchyma. It may also be referred to as a nephroblastoma and occurs in pediatric patients, usually between the ages of 1 and 5 years. (Moss et al., 1992, p.968)
32. (b) Ethmoid sinus (Lane and Sharfaei, 1992, p.71)
33. (a) The section thickness of a CT scan directly affects the detail and spatial resolution of the image. Narrow section widths result in greater detail when imaging small anatomic parts such as the sinuses. (Seeram, 1994, p.202)
34. (d) Number 2 corresponds to the zygomatic bone. (Lane and Sharfaei, 1992, p.71)
35. (d) Owing to their relatively high CT numbers, gallstones usually appear hyperdense when compared with the bile-filled gallbladder. Some gallstones having lower attenuation values can appear isodense on a CT scan of the abdomen. (Moss et al., 1992, p.840)
36. (a) Subdural hematomas caused by relatively recent trauma appear as hyperdense areas on CT images of the brain. Intravenous iodinated contrast media are not necessary for their visualization and may act to conceal them. Contrast media are extremely valuable for visualization of intracranial tumors. (Putman and Ravin, 1994, p.188)
37. (c) Left common iliac vein (Chiu et al., 1995, p.143)
38. (c) Portions of the CT image may be enlarged on the display screen by either of two methods. The image may be magnified, offering the

viewer a closer, enlarged look at a specific area, or a CT image may be "targeted" through a decrease in the DFOV size. A targeted image places the region of interest over the entire display matrix, providing increased resolution and detail over a magnified image. (Berland, 1987, p.81)

39. (b) Right ureter (Chiu et al., 1995, p.143)
40. (d) Rectus abdominis muscle (Chiu et al., 1995, p.143)
41. (d) Axial images of the neck are easily programmed from a lateral projection scanogram or scout. (Berland, 1987, p.216)
42. (d) The acetabulum is a cup-shaped cavity that holds the head of the femur, forming the hip joint. It is composed of portions of the ilium, ischium, and pubis. (Clemente, 1985, p.269)
43. (b) Pedicle (Wicke, 1994, p.232)
44. (a) CT images of the spine are commonly reconstructed using small DFOV sizes within the range of 12–15 cm. DFOVs within this range reconstruct the spine in an enlarged fashion while maintaining good detail. (Berland, 1987, p.47)
45. (d) Costovertebral articulation (Wicke, 1994, p.232)
46. (c) Descending aorta (Wicke, 1994, p.232)
47. (b) The pancreas is a common area for CT-guided needle biopsies. The location of a pathologic process and the type of tissue involved govern the use of percutaneous biopsy under CT guidance. (Lee et al., 1989, p.97)
48. (d) Diatrizoate meglumine is an ionic intravenous contrast material, whereas iopamidol is a non-ionic one. Both may be used for soft-tissue enhancement during CT of the chest. A barium sulfate contrast, usually in the form of a paste, may also be used to outline the esophagus. (Katzberg, 1992, p.5; p.192)
49. (c) Pulmonary hilum (Moss et al., 1992, p.121)
50. (b) CT scans are often performed for radiation therapy treatment planning. These scans localize an area of malignant pathology so that radiation treatments may be precisely given. During this type of specialized CT scan, the patient must be positioned in the exact same position that will be used during the radiation treatments. This includes using a hard, flat tabletop that mimics the one used in radiation therapy. A flat board or table insert is used to create a surface similar to that used during radiation therapy. (Berland, 1987, p.244)
51. (b) Number 2 most likely corresponds to a tumor. (Moss et al., 1992, p.132)
52. (d) The pituitary gland produces several hormones, including somatotropin and prolactin. It is the adrenal glands that play a role in the production and secretion of epinephrine (adrenaline). (Clemente, 1985, p.1600)

53. (c) General survey CT studies for lymphoma may be performed with spacings of 15–20 mm when using an aperture size of 10 mm. Contiguous scans may be performed on specific areas. (Berland, 1987, p.237)
54. (b) Number 3 corresponds to the trapezius muscle. (Bo et al., 1990, p.44)
55. (c) A total contrast volume between 100 and 150 mL is sufficient when imaging the neck. The precise volume and the administration technique vary among institutions. (Berland, 1987, p.216)
56. (a) Common carotid artery (Bo et al., 1990, p.44)
57. (d) Levator scapulae muscle (Bo et al., 1990, p.44)
58. (d) The kidneys are located in a portion of the retroperitoneum known as Gerota's space. They are held in place by fibrous connective tissue commonly referred to as Gerota's fascia. (Gedgaudas-McClees and Torres, 1990, p.27)
59. (b) Dynamic CT scans are those obtained at a rapid pace with minimized interscan delays. These types of CT examinations are usually done in conjunction with the intravenous administration of iodinated contrast media. The rapid-sequence scanning allows for data acquisition during the peak enhancement phase, taking full advantage of the attenuation-altering contrast material. (Berland, 1987, p.206)
60. (a) The coronal plane divides the body into anterior and posterior portions. This section has been obtained from the dorsal surface through the plantar surface of the foot, with the anterior portion removed. (Ballinger, 1995, p.49)
61. (a) First metatarsal (Firooznia et al., 1992, p.862)
62. (c) Sesamoid bones (Clemente, 1985, p.304)
63. (a) A solution of 2%–5% iodinated water-soluble contrast and water provides sufficient bowel opacification for CT studies of the abdomen and pelvis. Some institutions may use flavored contrast or add a flavoring agent to the solution for ease of consumption. Common water-soluble contrast media include Gastrografin and Hypaque. (Katzberg, 1992, p.202)
64. (c) Number 1 corresponds to the superior mesenteric vein. (Chiu et al., 1995, p.125)
65. (b) Spleen (Chiu et al., 1995, p.125)
66. (d) Pancreas (Chiu et al., 1995, p.125)
67. (c) The patient is usually placed in the supine position, head first into the gantry for a CT examination of the brain. (Seeram, 1994, p.269)
68. (b) A sagittally reformatted image would demonstrate the relationship of the disk material as it protrudes posteriorly onto the spinal cord. (Seeram, 1994, p.172)
69. (d) Low spatial frequency algorithms are usually referred to as standard or soft-tissue algorithms. They filter out high spatial frequency

information, such as that pertaining to bone, and provide maximum detail of soft-tissue structures. (Seeram, 1994, p.202)

70. (a) Interstitial diseases of the lungs are usually diffuse pathologic processes involving the interstitium, or framework, of the lungs. Examples of interstitial diseases include bronchiectasis, emphysema, asbestosis, and sarcoidosis. (Moss et al., 1992, p.166)
71. (c) The high-density object leading from the skin surface into the pancreatic head indicates that this image is part of a CT-guided needle biopsy. (Gedgaudas-McClees and Torres, 1990, p.268)
72. (d) Biopsy needle (Chiu et al., 1995, p.198)
73. (d) Gallbladder (Bo et al., 1990, p.136)
74. (c) Stomach (Bo et al., 1990, p.136)
75. (d) Cerebrospinal fluid is produced and secreted by the choroid plexuses that are located in each of the four ventricles of the brain. (Guyton, 1986, p.375)
76. (b) Small amounts of gas may appear in the areas of degenerated intervertebral disks. The accumulation of gases such as nitrogen occurs as a by-product of the physical breakdown of the disk material. (Lee et al., 1989, p.997)
77. (c) The hip joint is located at the same level as the greater trochanter of the femur and the pubic bone. Palpation of either of these areas should be used to accurately center the hip within the gantry. (Ballinger, 1995, p.40)
78. (c) Ischium (Bo et al., 1990, p.206)
79. (d) Number 2 corresponds to the acetabulum. (Bo et al., 1990, p.206)
80. (a) Pubis (Bo et al., 1990, p.206)
81. (c) Stereotactic biopsy units are localization devices designed specifically for CT-guided biopsies. They are most commonly used for intercranial lesions because precision and accuracy are extremely important. (Berland, 1987, p.121)
82. (c) Intravenous iodinated contrast administration is vital in making an accurate diagnosis of a dissecting aortic aneurysm. The contrast helps to outline the wall of the aorta and improves visualization of any division within it. Also, the CT numbers within the actual lumen of the aorta are different from those of the dissected portion owing to differences in blood flow. (Moss et al., 1992, p.72)
83. (b) Esophagus (Bo et al., 1990, p.206)
84. (c) Clavicle (Bo et al., 1990, p.206)
85. (d) Thyroid gland (Bo et al., 1990, p.206)
86. (c) The thyroid gland is significantly enlarged. This may be due to several processes, including thyroid carcinoma and various endocrine disorders. (Moss et al., 1992, p.410)
87. (d) Double-contrast CT examinations are valuable for the evaluation of the bladder. A Foley catheter is inserted into the bladder for the

direct administration of 100–300 mL of air and 100 mL of diluted diatrizoate meglumine. The contrast solution should consist of approximately 30% diatrizoate meglumine. (Moss et al., 1992, p.1184)

88. (d) The intervertebral disk spaces of a patient with severe lateral scoliosis may be difficult to evaluate. Placing the patient in a lateral decubitus position and angling the gantry through the disk spaces should improve visualization. (Lee et al., 1989, p.990)
89. (c) Psoas major muscle (Bo et al., 1990, p.136)
90. (b) Region of interest or attenuation measurements may be made on the CT image through numerous software applications. The image shown has a circular cursor positioned over an area of the kidney. The computer is capable of calculating the average attenuation value (CT number) for the pixels included within the circle. This information is valuable in determining the type of tissue present and can aid in the determination of a diagnosis for selected pathologic conditions. (Berland, 1987, p.107)
91. (d) The diagnosis of a renal cyst from a CT scan depends on several factors. The area must be of relatively homogeneous density with explicit demarcations from the surrounding renal tissue. It must also present no remarkable enhancement after intravenous contrast administration, maintaining an average Hounsfield value of zero (±20 Hounsfield units). (Gedgaudas-McClees and Torres, 1990, p.144)
92. (b) CT examinations for the evaluation of renal cysts should be performed before and after contrast administration to determine whether the region of interest enhances. A renal cyst should also have an average density near or equal to that of water: −20 to +20 Hounsfield units. (Berland, 1987, p.236)
93. (c) Liver (Bo et al., 1990, p.136)
94. (a) The seminal vesicles are located posterior to the bladder and anterior to the rectum on a cross section of the male pelvis. (Moss et al., 1992, p.1187)
95. (c) A scout or scanogram for a CT examination of the chest should be a frontal projection including from above the apices to just below the costophrenic angles. The patient's arms should be positioned overhead to avoid streaking artifacts. (Chiu et al., 1995, p.83)
96. (a) Acromion (Wicke, 1994, p.82)
97. (c) Carina (Clemente, 1985, p.1378)
98. (b) Costophrenic angle (Wicke, 1994, p.82)
99. (c) The prone position during a post-myelographic CT study of the lumbar spine reduces pooling or layering of the intrathecal contrast material. (Lee et al., 1989, p.990)
100. (a) The cul-de-sac is the area posterior to the uterus and ovaries in the female patient. It is a common site for ascites in the patient with pelvic disease. (Putman and Ravin, 1994, p.2018)

101. (b) Number 2 corresponds to the lateral rectus muscle. (Chiu et al., 1995, p.65)
102. (d) Ethmoid sinus (Chiu et al., 1995, p.65)
103. (c) The image includes the anatomic areas of the paranasal sinuses and the orbits. (Chiu et al., 1995, p.48)
104. (c) Optic nerve (Clemente, 1985, p.1306)
105. (b) Nasal bone (Chiu et al., 1995, p.65)

C. Physics and Instrumentation

106. (a) The x-ray beam of a first-generation CT scanner was highly collimated to the size of a single detector. It was often referred to as a "pencil beam." (Seeram, 1994, p.88)
107. (c) Blood has an approximate CT number value of +45 Hounsfield units. (Wolbarst, 1993, p.321)
108. (b) The analog-to-digital converter transforms the "analog" signal from the detectors into a numeric form that can be used by the computer. Analog information is based on a scale, whereas digital information is in numeric form. (Seeram, 1994, p.14)
109. (b) The pixel is a two-dimensional representation of a voxel. The section width is equal to the length of the voxel. To calculate the dimensions of a voxel, the pixel dimension must be multiplied by the section width. (Seeram, 1994, p.80)
110. (c) The attenuation coefficient of a tissue describes the ability of the tissue to attenuate x-radiation. CT numbers are assigned to pixels based on the attenuation of the tissue within the voxel. The assignment of a CT number in Hounsfield units arises from a comparison of the attenuation coefficient of the tissue to that of water. Materials with attenuation coefficients less than that of water are assigned negative CT numbers. (Wolbarst, 1993, p.321)
111. (d) The ability of a CT scanner to image objects with similar densities accurately is termed contrast resolution or sensitivity. A CT scanner with poor contrast resolution or low sensitivity has difficulty separating tissues whose linear attenuation coefficients are nearly equal. (Seeram, 1994, p.206)
112. (d) Large aperture sizes result in long voxel lengths with possibly several tissue types accounted for within the voxel. When a CT number is assigned to the representative pixel, the densities of all of the tissue types are averaged, yielding one attenuation coefficient. Narrow section widths tend to decrease the partial volume effect. (Berland, 1987, p.159)
113. (b) The spatial resolution of a CT image is dependent upon several factors, including focal spot size, detector size and spacing, field of view, pixel dimension, matrix size, and detector sampling rate. (Moss et al., 1992, p.1370)

114. (c) Retrospective reconstruction occurs when an image is reconstructed a second time with an adjustment in a technical factor. The scan data (or "raw" data) are used to reconstruct the image with different parameters (e.g., display matrix, DFOV, algorithm). (Berland, 1987, p.83)
115. (d) Cupping artifacts occur when the periphery of an image is much higher in density than the center. This difference in density causes beam hardening to affect the accuracy of the image negatively. The dense bone that surrounds the soft tissue of the brain is a common site for cupping artifacts to occur. (Berland, 1987, p.96)
116. (d) The matrix size used to reconstruct an image can be calculated by dividing the DFOV by the pixel dimension. A pixel whose area is 0.25 mm^2 has a linear dimension of 0.5 mm. The DFOV of 250 mm is divided by the pixel dimension of 0.5 mm, giving a matrix size of approximately 512 $\times$ 512 pixels. (Seeram, 1994, p.79)
117. (b) CT scanners are often placed into one of five different "generations." The different generations are based on the relationship of the tube and detectors and the position of each during data acquisition. (Seeram, 1994, p.87)
118. (c) The quantum or statistical noise of a CT image can be reduced by increasing the number of x-ray photons absorbed by the detectors for each voxel of tissue. This can be accomplished with increases in technique (mAs) and increases in the pixel and voxel dimensions. (Seeram, 1994, p.211)
119. (b) The first-generation prototype CT scanner designed by Dr. Godfrey Hounsfield used an iterative form of image reconstruction. (Seeram, 1994, p.133)
120. (b) The width of a window determines the range of pixel values assigned a shade of gray around a given level. In this example, all pixels within the range of −250 and +250 Hounsfield units will be assigned shades of gray. Pixels with values less than −250 Hounsfield units will appear black, and pixels with values more than +250 Hounsfield units will appear white. (Berland, 1987, p.123)
121. (c) Maximum intensity projections (MIPs) are commonly used during specialized studies such as CT angiography. An MIP image is constructed by displaying only the maximum intensity pixel found along each ray. A ray is the path from the focal spot of the x-ray tube to a detector. This technique is valuable in displaying contrast-enhanced blood vessels that are surrounded by various types of tissue. (Fishman and Brooke, 1995, p.171)
122. (b) The spatial resolution of a CT scanner controls its ability to image small structures. (Seeram, 1994, p.202)
123. (d) Although the CT technologist must be able to identify them readily, ring artifacts are caused by detector malfunction and are

beyond the technologist's control. Patient motion, partial volume averaging, and edge gradient artifacts can all be limited by the CT technologist through adequate preparation and careful scan procedures. (Curry et al., 1990, p.320)

124. (b) Quality control tests for CT number accuracy and noise levels should be performed daily on CT scanners. The laser localization system of a CT scanner needs to be checked only once per year. (Seeram, 1994, p.235)
125. (b) Increases in filtration cause a greater amount of low-energy x-ray photons to be absorbed, thereby increasing the average photon energy of the beam. Increases in mAs increase the intensity of the beam but do not affect average photon energy. (Seeram, 1994, p.96)
126. (c) Streaking artifacts commonly occur during CT scanning of thick body parts such as the shoulder. The x-ray beam changes in quality as it passes through different densities. These beam energy changes sometimes manifest themselves as streak artifacts. (Berland, 1987, p.153)
127. (a) High spatial frequency algorithms demonstrate the greatest spatial resolution and are best suited for imaging sharp density changes such as those occurring with bone tissue. "Bone," "edge," and "detail" are names commonly given to high spatial frequency algorithms. (Seeram, 1994, p.205)
128. (d) The window level used to display an image should equal the average Hounsfield value of the tissue of interest. In this example, the demonstration of bone tissue is most important. The type of bone making up the shoulder joint would have an average density of +250 Hounsfield units. (Berland, 1987, p.127)
129. (b) The greatest disruptor of contrast resolution is noise. Noise appears as a graininess that can obscure the outline and delineation of structures, thus limiting the ability of the scanner to separate them. (Berland, 1987, p.91)
130. (c) CT images are usually constructed from transmission data acquired during a 360° rotation of the x-ray tube. A CT image can also be constructed from a portion of the data acquisition phase. For example, if a patient moves during the last third of a 2-second scan, an image can be constructed from the first 240° of tube rotation, yielding an image free of motion. This process is referred to as segmentation and is a software capability of many modern CT scanners. (Berland, 1987, p.119)
131. (b) Reference detectors are used to measure incident radiation intensity. This information is used by the computer during the calculation of the linear attenuation coefficient. If the patient is placed incorrectly within the gantry, the reference detectors may be partially blocked, causing an out-of-field artifact. (Berland, 1987, p.155)

132. (c) The edge gradient effect occurs at areas of abrupt change in density, which are represented by high spatial frequency signal. The computer may have difficulty interpreting this type of rapidly changing information, and streaks may appear as a result. The interface between dense bone and soft tissue is a common site for the edge gradient effect to occur. (Berland, 1987, p.149)
133. (d) Both the x-ray tube and the detector array rotate around the patient during scanning with a third-generation CT unit. (Seeram, 1994, p.89)
134. (d) The modulation transfer function (MTF) is a mathematical method of quantifying the spatial resolution of a CT scanner. (Seeram, 1994, p.198)
135. (a) The edge gradient artifact manifests itself as a streaking effect at areas of extremely high density interfaces. (Berland, 1987, p.149)
136. (c) High-density objects such as surgical clips and other types of prosthetic devices are often the cause of streaking artifacts due to the edge gradient effect. (Berland, 1987, p.156)
137. (b) The DFOV chosen for an image should be large enough to include the entire region of interest. (Berland, 1987, p.47)
138. (c) Dr. Godfrey Hounsfield and Dr. Allan Cormack shared the Nobel Prize for their work on the development of CT in 1979. (Seeram, 1994, p.8)
139. (b) The contrast of a CT image is controlled by the spatial frequencies of the tissues within the section. Tissues of differing densities are represented electronically by different spatial frequencies. Adjacent tissues with large differences in density are represented by high spatial frequency signal. (Berland, 1987, p.33)
140. (d) The dimensions of a pixel may be calculated by dividing the DFOV by the matrix size. The pixel is a square with four equal sides, and the dimension of one side is usually given in millimeters. The area of the pixel is calculated by squaring the dimension, and the units are then adjusted to millimeters squared (mm^2). (Seeram, 1994, p.80)
141. (a) The bit is the smallest unit of information within the binary system. Its name is derived from the "binary digit," and it can appear as either a number 1 or 0. A sequence of eight bits constitutes a byte. (Wolbarst, 1993, p.300)
142. (d) The CT number of a pixel may be calculated by subtracting the linear attenuation coefficient of water from the linear attenuation coefficient of the tissue within the voxel. This number is then divided by the linear attenuation coefficient of water. The quotient is then multiplied by a scaling factor of 1000 to yield the value of the pixel in Hounsfield units. (Seeram, 1994, p.74)
143. (c) The transmitted intensity is the amount of energy that passes through the patient onto a detector. (Seeram, 1994, p.71)

144. (d) The purpose of predetector (or postpatient) collimation is to remove scatter radiation and to shape the portion of the beam that reaches each detector. (Seeram, 1994, p.98)
145. (b) Metallic items such as dental fillings are a common cause of streaking or "star" artifact. (Berland, 1987, p.156)
146. (b) The only effective method of reducing streak artifact caused by metal is to remove the metal objects from the scanning field. In this case, the dental fillings cannot be removed, but the gantry could be angled to avoid their interference. (Berland, 1987, p.156)
147. (a) The pixel dimension may be calculated by dividing the DFOV by the matrix size. This two-dimensional pixel size is then multiplied by the length of the voxel. (Seeram, 1994, p.80)
148. (c) The quantum noise of a CT image can be reduced with an increase in the number of x-ray photons reaching the detectors. This may be accomplished with an increase in mAs or an increase in section width (decreased collimation). (Seeram, 1994, p.211)
149. (c) Referred to as "targeting," decreases in the DFOV cause an increase in the image size on the monitor. The DFOV controls the amount of scanned information to be displayed on the monitor. If a small portion of information is to be displayed on the entire matrix, it will appear larger in size to the viewer. (Berland, 1987, p.84)
150. (b) The minimum object size that a CT scanner can resolve may be calculated by taking the reciprocal value of the limiting resolution of the scanner. The reciprocal of 15 lp/cm is 1/15 lp/cm. This is equivalent to 10/15 lp/mm, which equals 0.6 mm/lp. Because a line pair (lp) is equivalent to a line and the space adjacent to it, this value may be divided in half to provide the minimum object that this scanner can resolve: 0.3 mm. (Seeram, 1994, p.198)

CHAPTER 8

Answer Key for Simulated Exam Four

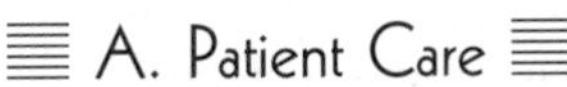

A. Patient Care

1. (c) The normal range for pulse rate in a child is 70–120 beats per minute. This is slightly faster than the rate of 60–100 beats per minute for an adult. (Adler and Carlton, 1994, p.181)
2. (c) Hypovolemic shock is caused by an insufficient volume of circulating blood. The common signs and symptoms of hypovolemic shock include pallor (absence of color in the skin), hypotension, tachycardia, and oliguria (decreased urine production). (Torres, 1993, p.91)
3. (b) Common sites for intravenous contrast injection include the antecubital, basilic, cephalic, and accessory cephalic veins. Intra-arterial injections of contrast material are not routinely performed for CT examinations. The only exceptions occur during hepatic CT angiography, when contrast may be administered through a catheter placed in either the superior mesenteric artery or the celiac artery. (Katzberg, 1992, p.69)
4. (c) Many CT scanners allow the technologist to reduce the total rotation of the x-ray tube, thus reducing the scan time and subsequent patient dose. This type of application is commonly referred to as a partial scan or "half-scan." (Berland, 1987, p.66)
5. (b) Parenteral routes of medication administration include intramuscular, intravenous, intradermal, and subcutaneous. (Torres, 1993, p.213)
6. (d) The viscosity of a contrast material can be reduced by heating it to body temperature (98.6°F/37°C). The decrease in viscosity allows for easier administration of the contrast material. (Katzberg, 1992, p.6)
7. (d) Examples of mild adverse reactions to iodinated contrast material include nausea, vomiting, mild urticaria, and a warm, flushed sensation.

Dyspnea is a moderate reaction, whereas pulmonary edema and shock are severe reactions to contrast media. (Putman and Ravin, 1994, p.1068)

8. (a) The patient is required to provide informed consent before the start of any invasive procedure. A noncontrast CT study of the brain is not invasive and therefore does not require informed consent. (Adler and Carlton, 1994, p.350)
9. (c) Non-ionic contrast media include iopamidol (Isovue), iohexol (Omnipaque), and iopromide (Ultravist). (Carr, 1988, p.7)
10. (a) The top number of a blood pressure measurement is the systolic pressure. This is a measure of the pressure exerted on the arterial walls during a contraction of the heart. (Adler and Carlton, 1994, p.185)
11. (c) Epinephrine (Adrenalin) is an adrenergic drug used as a bronchodilator. Diphenhydramine (Benadryl) may be used to block the physiologic effects of the release of histamine, thus reducing the allergic effect of the contrast. Atropine should be used only to combat bradycardia during a vagal reaction to contrast. (Katzberg, 1992, p.24)
12. (b) The osmolality of a contrast material is a measure of the number of particles per kilogram of water. Osmolality is a factor in determining the potential for adverse reaction from iodinated contrast material. Non-ionic contrast media have an average osmolality of 750 mOsm/kg of water. When compared with ionic media, a non-ionic contrast agent dissociates into fewer particles. Ionic contrast media have an average osmolality of 1000–2400 mOsm/kg. (Tortorici and Apfel, 1995, p.21)
13. (b) An autoclave is a mechanical device used for sterilization. It involves the use of heat and steam under pressure to eliminate microbes. An oven uses only high heat and is not as efficient as an autoclave. (Adler and Carlton, 1994, p.208)
14. (c) The partial thromboplastin time is a laboratory measure of blood coagulation. This value is used to screen patients for invasive procedures. Due to variations in individual laboratory practices, the average range may fluctuate slightly. (*The Merck Manual*, 1987, p.1153)
15. (d) Gonadal shielding may be used whenever the gonads do not lie within the region of clinical interest. Gonadal shielding in the female patient is most difficult during CT scanning of the pelvis. (Berland, 1987, p.42)
16. (c) An immediate alert should be initiated at the beginning of cardiopulmonary resuscitation. This involves a call for help from coworkers or the appropriate emergency staff. (Adler and Carlton, 1994, p.263)
17. (a) In order for a suction unit to properly drain a chest tube, it must always remain below the level of the patient. (Torres, 1993, p.157)
18. (d) The flow rate may be calculated by dividing the total contrast volume by the time of the injection. In this example, the total contrast

volume is 125 mL and the time for the injection is 50 seconds. The flow rate programmed for this injection is 2.5 mL/sec. (Snopek, 1992, p.49)

19. (c) An ionization chamber is a device used to accurately measure radiation exposure. Radiation causes ionization within the chamber, which is measured by an electrode. The amount of ionization within the chamber is proportional to the radiation exposure. This is an extremely accurate device that is used to quantify radiation exposure from a CT scan. (Seeram, 1994, p.221)
20. (d) Although not an absolute contraindication to intravenous contrast administration, an allergic history to shellfish may warrant the use of non-ionic contrast material. Intravenous contrast should not be administered to patients with acute sickle cell anemia, pheochromocytoma, or an elevated serum creatinine level. (Katzberg, 1992, p.71)
21. (a) The patient should have nothing by mouth (NPO) for several hours before a contrast-enhanced CT examination of the chest. This reduces the incidence of nausea, vomiting, and possible aspiration of contrast material. (Berland, 1987, p.199)
22. (a) The multiple-scan average dose (MSAD) is used to quantify the amount of exposure a patient receives from a series of CT scans. The MSAD is calculated from the CT dose index (CTDI) through a series of equations. The quantity of radiation per scan is measured using an ionization chamber. (Seeram, 1994, p.222)
23. (c) The contrast medium iohexol (Omnipaque) is a recently developed non-ionic contrast agent that may be used for intrathecal injection. Other types of intrathecal contrast media include metrizamide (Amipaque) and iopamidol (Isovue). (Firooznia et al., 1992, p.131)
24. (a) Larger-gauge needles allow for more-rapid intravenous administration of contrast media. The lumen is considerably larger in a 19-gauge needle than in a 25-gauge needle. The viscosity of contrast material necessitates the use of a relatively large-bore needle. (Katzberg, 1992, p.75)
25. (a) It is important to be aware of the serum creatinine level of a patient scheduled to undergo a postcontrast CT examination. This is especially true for any patient with a history of renal disease. The serum creatinine level is a laboratory value used to measure renal function, and abnormally elevated values are often signs of renal failure. (Laudicina and Wean, 1994, p.32)
26. (d) A faint or lightheaded feeling is commonly referred to as syncope. (*Mosby's Medical Dictionary,* 1994)
27. (c) Enteric precautions attempt to protect from the spread of infection through direct or indirect contact with fecal matter. Gowns and gloves are common protective attire used for enteric precautions. The use of a surgical mask is not warranted. (Torres, 1993, p.39)

28. (b) The coagulation capabilities of a patient may be evaluated with the measurement of prothrombin time and partial thromboplastin time. Each of these laboratory values attempts to detect deficiencies in the various blood clotting factors. Hematocrit is the concentration of red blood cells within the total volume of blood. It may be used to evaluate the hydration status of a patient. (Laudicina and Wean, 1994, p.32)
29. (d) None of these indwelling catheters or central venous lines should be used for the injection of contrast material with a power injector. Only the Hickman catheter can be reasonably used for nondynamic injections of contrast material. The pressure applied by an automatic injector is too great to be withstood by these types of long-term lines. (Katzberg, 1992, p.75)
30. (b) A bolus administration of contrast material requires the entire volume of material to be injected over the shortest possible time. Accomplished by hand or with the use of an automatic injector, bolus administration provides the maximum plasma–iodine concentration and subsequent tissue enhancement. (Katzberg, 1992, p.68)

B. Imaging Procedures

31. (c) High-resolution CT is a specialized technique using narrow section widths and a high-resolution algorithm for image reconstruction. It is used to maximize detail of high spatial frequency tissue such as the lungs and bony structures. (Moss et al., 1992, p.157)
32. (b) Lidocaine is a common local anesthetic used for preparation of the needle insertion site during a percutaneous biopsy. (Lee et al., 1989, p.92)
33. (a) Greater trochanter (Clemente, 1985, p.275)
34. (c) The image quality of three-dimensional reconstructed images is greatly improved with the use of narrow, overlapping sections. This increases the total volume of information used to construct the three-dimensional model. The use of a small scan field of view (SFOV) in the area of the hip would cause an out-of-field artifact. (Seeram, 1994, p.252)
35. (c) Ilium (Clemente, 1985, p.270)
36. (d) Femoral neck (Clemente, 1985, p.275)
37. (d) Number 3 corresponds to the ischium (Clemente, 1985, p.273)
38. (c) The density of the liver greatly decreases with the presence of fatty infiltrates. The minimal attenuation of fat and its low CT number cause an overall decrease in the attenuation and CT number of the hepatic parenchyma. (Gedgaudas-McClees and Torres, 1990, p.94)
39. (a) Number 3 corresponds to the left retromandibular vein. (Bo et al., 1990, p.38)

40. (c) A contiguous study with an aperture size ranging from 3–6 mm is sufficient for a general survey CT study of the neck. (Berland, 1987, p.218)
41. (b) Oropharynx (Bo et al., 1990, p.38)
42. (c) Pharyngeal constrictor muscle (Bo et al., 1990, p.42)
43. (c) The thymus gland may be found in the anterosuperior portion of the mediastinum. It is most easily visible in patients before puberty. After the patient reaches puberty, the thymus gland becomes increasingly infiltrated with fat, making it more difficult to image with CT. (Lee et al., 1989, p.213)
44. (c) Falciform ligament (Bo et al., 1990, p.130)
45. (d) Caudate lobe of the liver (Bo et al., 1990, p.130)
46. (c) CT examinations of the abdomen usually include the administration of both oral and intravenous iodinated contrast media. The administration of oral effervescent negative contrast would cause marked distension of the stomach. This is not evident in Figure 4–3, in which the walls of the stomach appear thickened and the stomach is not inflated with gas. (Moss et al., 1992, p.660)
47. (d) Gastric rugae (Moss et al., 1992, p.660)
48. (b) Right crus of diaphragm (Bo et al., 1990, p.126)
49. (c) Due to their increased CT number, subdural hematomas may be well visualized without the administration of intravenous iodinated contrast. (Chiu et al., 1995, p.23)
50. (c) The window width used to provide maximum detail of bony structures is approximately 1200 to 2000 Hounsfield units. This relatively wide width allows for complete visualization of the variable densities present in bony anatomic areas. (Berland, 1987, p.213)
51. (d) Sacral foramen (Clemente, 1985, p.141)
52. (c) The pathologic process shown in the figure is a fractured sacrum. Note the interruption in the smooth delineation of the right anterior sacrum. (Firooznia et al., 1992, p.417)
53. (b) Contrast enhancement is at its lowest point during the equilibrium phase. This phase is apparent when the aorta and inferior vena cava differ by less than 10 Hounsfield units. It is during this phase that hepatic lesions may become isodense with the surrounding hepatic parenchyma. Noncontrast scanning of the liver is actually preferred to scanning during the equilibrium phase. (Katzberg, 1992, p.68)
54. (b) The CT technologist is often asked to localize the exact area of the kidneys. Although there may be some fluctuation from patient to patient, the kidneys can usually be found between the twelfth thoracic vertebra and the third lumbar vertebra. (Moss et al., 1992, p.942)
55. (a) Right brachiocephalic vein (Bo et al., 1990, p.78)
56. (d) Left common carotid artery (Bo et al., 1990, p.78)
57. (c) Brachiocephalic artery (Bo et al., 1990, p.78)

58. (d) Number 1 corresponds to the left brachiocephalic vein. (Bo et al., 1990, p.78)
59. (a) The subclavian, brachiocephalic, and common carotid arteries branch off the superior portion of the aortic arch. The left and right brachiocephalic veins originate from the superior vena cava. (Clemente, 1985, p.628)
60. (b) This technique allows for visualization of the relationship between the patella and the femur as the knee is increasingly flexed. The patellofemoral congruence, or the position of the patella within the patella surface of the femur, may be measured at each point of flexion. Any medial or lateral displacement of the patella may indicate an abnormality of the patellofemoral joint. (Firooznia et al., 1992, p.666)
61. (a) Right common iliac vein (Bo et al., 1990, p.152)
62. (c) Psoas muscle (Bo et al., 1990, p.152)
63. (b) Iliac crest (Bo et al., 1990, p.152)
64. (c) The iliac crest may be used as a landmark to locate the level of the fourth lumbar vertebra. (Ballinger, 1995, p.40)
65. (d) Number 1 corresponds to the left common iliac artery. (Bo et al., 1990, p.152)
66. (c) Ascending colon (Bo et al., 1990, p.152)
67. (b) The easiest patient position for the acquisition of this localizer image is supine with the knees flexed and the plantar portion of the foot placed in contact with the table. (Firooznia et al., 1992, p.821)
68. (a) Navicular (Ballinger, 1995, p.198)
69. (b) Cuboid (Ballinger, 1995, p.198)
70. (b) Talus (Ballinger, 1995, p.201)
71. (b) The tarsals include the calcaneus, talus, navicular, cuboid, and medial, intermediate, and lateral cuneiforms. (Ballinger, 1995, p.180)
72. (c) The coronal plane divides the body into anterior and posterior portions. CT scans perpendicular to the scout image in Figure 4–7 provide coronal images when the body is considered in anatomic position. (Firooznia et al., 1992, p.821)
73. (c) The total length of the scan may be calculated by multiplying the scan time by the aperture size. In this example, the scan time is 15 seconds with an aperture size (section thickness) of 1.0 cm or 10 mm. At the end of this scan, a total volume of 150 mm of the pelvis will have been imaged. (Fishman and Brooke, 1995, p.2)
74. (d) CT images of the brain should be acquired parallel to the skull base. Placing the patient in the supine position with the chin down facilitates the axial acquisition at an angle 15° above the orbitomeatal line. (Chiu et al., 1995, p.21)
75. (c) Third ventricle (Chiu et al., 1995, p.31)
76. (b) Vermis of cerebellum (Bo et al., 1990, p.14)
77. (b) Putamen (Chiu et al., 1995, p.33)

78. (c) Thalamus (Bo et al., 1990, p.12)
79. (a) Number 6 corresponds to the genu of corpus callosum. (Bo et al., 1990, p.10)
80. (b) When one views cross-sectional anatomy, the image should be oriented with the left side of the patient on the right side of the viewer with a perspective up from the feet toward the head. (Seeram, 1994, p.264)
81. (b) An acoustic neuroma (schwannoma) arises from Schwann cells of the eighth cranial nerve, or the vestibulocochlear nerve. This type of cranial mass may be imaged with CT examinations of the internal auditory canals. (Putman and Ravin, 1994, p.215)
82. (b) Lamina (Chiu et al., 1995, p.164)
83. (d) A useful guide to ensure complete coverage of a lumbar disk is to scan from the pedicle of the vertebra above to the pedicle of the vertebra below the disk. (Lee et al., 1989, p.993)
84. (a) Number 1 corresponds to the pedicle. (Chiu et al., 1995, p.164)
85. (b) Intrathecal iodinated contrast allows for greater visualization of the spinal cord and nerve roots after its introduction into the subarachnoid space. (Chiu et al., 1995, p.162)
86. (d) Spinous process (Chiu et al., 1995, p.164)
87. (a) Dynamic scanning is accomplished with the shortest interscan delay possible. This type of CT scan takes maximum advantage of the tissue enhancement from a bolus administration of intravenous iodinated contrast. A CT unit may limit the amount of dynamic scans possible due to the limited heat capacity of most x-ray tubes. Spiral CT has begun to eliminate the need for dynamic CT due to its inherently rapid acquisition times. (Chiu et al., 1995, p.90)
88. (b) The localizer image used to program a CT scan of the abdomen should include from the area above the diaphragm to the level of the iliac crest. (Berland, 1987, p.228)
89. (c) The correlation feature of a CT scanner allows the outline of an anatomic area to be superimposed over a scout image. This provides a different perspective of the location and orientation of the area. (Berland, 1987, p.118)
90. (b) The left kidney has been correlated with the scout in the figure. The left kidney was outlined on the axial images with a cursor, and this information was then superimposed on the scout by the computer. (Berland, 1987, p.118)
91. (c) Left ventricle (Bo et al., 1990, p.106)
92. (d) The matrix size, algorithm, and section thickness can all be found on the peripheral portion of the image. Each of these factors is variable and greatly affects the image quality. (Lee et al., 1989, p.33)
93. (c) Azygos vein (Bo et al., 1990, p.106)

94. (b) The image was reconstructed in a display field of view (DFOV) larger than necessary. The image appears minified because of this error. The DFOV chosen for an image should be slightly larger than the diameter of the area of interest. The DFOV used here was 48 cm. This image would appear significantly larger with a DFOV of 36–40 cm. (Berland, 1987, p.47)
95. (d) The section shown in Figure 4–11 was obtained at a level below the left atrium. (Bo et al., 1990, p.106)
96. (d) Alzheimer's disease is not easily diagnosed from a CT scan of the brain. Some diagnostic differentiation may be found from enlargement of the temporal horns, but this is not specific on CT examinations. (Putman and Ravin, 1994, p.243)
97. (a) Most pancreatic tumors occur in the head of the pancreas. The majority of these masses are adenocarcinomas. (Gedgaudas-McClees and Torres, 1990, p.134)
98. (b) Number 7 corresponds to the gluteus medius muscle. (Bo et al., 1990, p.202)
99. (d) Femoral artery (Bo et al., 1990, p.202)
100. (c) Obturator internus muscle (Bo et al., 1990, p.202)
101. (b) Femoral vein (Bo et al., 1990, p.202)
102. (c) A delay of 45 seconds should be used when scanning the liver to allow the portal vein to become opacified. (Berland, 1987, p.209)
103. (d) MPR (multiplanar reformatted images) may be constructed in the coronal, sagittal, or any other transaxial plane. Computer manipulations allow the original axial acquisition to be volumetrically rotated and additional sections to be constructed. (Seeram, 1994, p.172)
104. (d) Roots of teeth (Ballinger, 1995, p.369)
105. (b) The reference image labeled as number 3 is an axial image of the mandible. (Seeram, 1994, p.172)

C. Physics and Instrumentation

106. (d) When the pitch is increased during a spiral CT scan, either the section width or the table speed has been increased. Any increase in section width will cause a subsequent increase in the partial volume effect. The increased table speed also plays a role in increasing partial volume averaging. As the table moves through the gantry at a faster rate, each rotation of the tube and detectors is responsible for recording more information. This causes a broadening of the section sensitivity profile, which manifests itself as partial volume averaging. (Fishman and Brooke, 1995, p.4)
107. (d) Misregistration is the loss of anatomic information that occurs when a patient suspends respiration at different depths during consecutive scans. It occurs only during CT examinations in which suspended respiration of the patient is necessary. (Berland, 1987, p.169)

108. (d) The point spread function (PSF), modulation transfer function (MTF), and line spread function (LSF) all are used to quantify the spatial resolution of a CT scanner. The LSF measures the ability of a CT scanner to clearly image an edge or line. The PSF does the same for extremely small point-like structures. The MTF examines the fidelity of the spatial frequency as it represents tissues with varying densities. The MTF is derived from the measurement of the LSF and PSF. (Seeram, 1994, p.198)
109. (b) Consisting of an arrangement of pixels in rows and columns, the matrix is used to organize the attenuation information from the anatomic section into a digital image. The size of the matrix is given as the number of pixels across multiplied by the number of pixels down. (Seeram, 1994, p.78)
110. (b) The iterative methods of CT image reconstruction include simultaneous reconstruction, ray by ray correction, and point by point correction. The Fourier transform method is an analytic method of CT image reconstruction. (Curry et al., 1990, p.305)
111. (c) The bow-tie filter used at the x-ray tube of a CT scanner absorbs a larger amount of radiation at the periphery of the patient where the part thickness is reduced. The center of the patient is placed at the center of the filter where the largest amount of radiation is allowed to pass through. The use of this type of filter attempts to compensate for the differences in thickness of the often oval patient. (Seeram, 1994, p.96)
112. (b) The Lambert-Beer law, $I = I_0e^{-\mu x}$, is used to calculate the attenuation coefficient of a volume of material. I_0 represents the intensity of the radiation incident on the tissue being imaged. It is compared with the intensity of the radiation passing through the tissue (I) during the calculation of the linear attenuation coefficient. (Seeram, 1994, p.70)
113. (b) A decrease in aperture size reduces the amount of x-ray photons exposing the tissue. This causes a decrease in the signal-to-noise ratio. The collimators used to adjust the size of the aperture absorb radiation as they restrict the beam. (Wolbarst, 1993, p.331)
114. (b) Computer programs are capable of constructing three-dimensional models of anatomy with several different types of rendering techniques. A surface-rendered three-dimensional model provides excellent surface anatomy appearance while maintaining the normal cross-sectional CT appearance of the volume inside the model. (Seeram, 1994, p.259)
115. (d) The computer software is able to remove quadrants of information to allow visualization of the inner portions of the model. In this example, the right anterior superior portion has been removed. This information can be ascertained by examining the anatomic position of

the model. On the image, the letters "RAS" signify "right anterior superior." (Seeram, 1994, p.176)

116. (a) In the Compton interaction, an x-ray photon ejects an outer shell electron of an atom. The photon loses some of its energy in the collision and then continues on in a different, scattered direction. This interaction is the major source of the scatter radiation involved in the formation of the CT image. (Curry et al., 1990, p. 65)

117. (c) The types of detectors used in CT include scintillation crystal and gas ionization detectors. Both operate by measuring the amount of transmitted radiation passed through the patient and transmitting this information to the computer for image reconstruction. (Seeram, 1994, p.99)

118. (c) VHS tape is a common video tape used to record dynamic images such as motion pictures from a video camera. CT images are digital static images that may be archived on floppy disk, magnetic tape, digital audio tape, and magnetic optical disk. (Berland, 1987, p.141)

119. (b) The test described is used to evaluate the cross-field uniformity of a CT scanner. The region of interest (ROI) measurements are arranged with one at the center of the image and the others rotated about the periphery. Each of the five ROI measurements taken from the water phantom should provide relatively the same CT number value. (Seeram, 1994, p.212)

120. (a) The adjustment of the window width or level is a computer manipulation of image data. The image has already been reconstructed from scan or "raw" data. The window changes only the range of pixel values that are assigned a shade of gray. Adjustments in the algorithm, DFOV, or matrix require the raw data so that the image may be retrospectively reconstructed. (Seeram, 1994, p.166)

121. (c) Collimation of the x-ray beam in CT consists of both prepatient collimators and predetector collimators. The prepatient collimator restricts the primary beam, thereby controlling the section thickness. The predetector or postpatient collimator absorbs scatter radiation before it contributes to the signal produced by the detector array. (Seeram, 1994, p.97)

122. (c) An average CT number value for bone is approximately +1000 Hounsfield units. This may vary widely with the density of the particular bone in question and with the beam quality of the CT scanner. (Wolbarst, 1993, p.321)

123. (b) The modulation transfer function (MTF) of a CT scanner measures the ability of the system to faithfully reproduce the area of anatomy. It can be thought of as a comparison of the actual anatomy to the image produced. If both are exactly alike, the MTF of the scanner has a value of 1. If the image produced contains no useful

information, the MTF value is 0. The MTF of most CT scanners usually falls somewhere in between. (Seeram, 1994, p.198)

124. (d) The star artifact was an unwanted by-product of the back-projection method of image reconstruction used in older CT scanners. The artifact is removed by the process of convolution used in the modern reconstruction method of filtered back-projection. (Seeram, 1994, p.130)
125. (b) Gases with high atomic numbers such as xenon are used in ionization-type CT detector systems. The high atomic number of the xenon gas (Z = 54) increases the incidence of interaction with x-ray photons, thus increasing the efficiency of the detector. (Curry et al., 1990, p.300)
126. (c) The most effective method of reducing involuntary motion on a CT scan is through reduced scan times. Many scanners offer "half-scan" options in which images may be reconstructed after a partial revolution of the tube–detector system. In the case of digestive involuntary motion, the additional option of glucagon administration exists. (Berland, 1987, p.163)
127. (a) CT images may be arranged in several different ways on a sheet of x-ray film. The format of the film pertains to the number and size of the images contained on each sheet. For example, a 4:1 format stores four large images on a single 14- × 17-inch film. A 15:1 format stores 15 smaller images on the same size film. (Seeram, 1994, p.157)
128. (c) Region of interest measurements may be made by superimposing a cursor over an area and instructing the computer to average the CT numbers included within the region. (Berland, 1987, p.107)
129. (c) The CT number for water has an average value of zero. (Wolbarst, 1993, p.321)
130. (d) A larger matrix size consists of an increased number of pixels. The computer is then able to assign less information into each pixel, allowing the image to display extremely small objects separately from one another. This increases the spatial resolution of the CT scanner. (Seeram, 1994, p.203)
131. (d) The data acquisition system of a CT scanner consists of the detector array, the analog-to-digital converter, and a transmission device used to send the converted digital information to the central processing unit for image reconstruction. (Seeram, 1994, p.103)
132. (b) An algorithm may be defined as a set of rules or steps used to solve a mathematical problem. The programs used by the CT computer to reconstruct the image are often referred to as algorithms. (Seeram, 1994, p.127)
133. (a) The contrast resolution of a CT scanner is dependent on several factors including section width, algorithm selection, detector sensitiv-

ity, and noise. The focal spot size is a geometric factor that influences the spatial resolution of a CT scanner. (Seeram, 1994, p.207)

134. (b) The spatial resolution of a scanner quantifies its ability to visually separate small objects in the image. The unit used to describe the spatial resolution of a CT scanner is line pairs per centimeter (lp/cm). Spatial resolution is tested by scanning a phantom with an embedded resolution test pattern consisting of a series of small lead lines that decrease in size and spacing. The smallest, most closely spaced set of lead lines is said to be the spatial resolution of the CT scanner. A line pair is one lead line and the space immediately next to it. (Seeram, 1994, p.198)
135. (c) The type of tissue included in a three-dimensional model may be limited by instructing the computer to include pixels with only a certain range of CT number values. Referred to as "thresholding," this technique is used to remove unwanted tissue types from a three-dimensional image, leaving only the tissue found within the threshold setting. (Seeram, 1994, p.254)
136. (c) A step artifact in a three-dimensional image occurs when the CT scan is performed with wide sections. When the three-dimensional model is produced, the delineation between consecutive sections may be seen. A reduction in section and width and the use of overlapping sections reduce the step artifact. (Seeram, 1994, p.259)
137. (d) Each CT scanner has several selections for SFOV. The SFOV selected by the technologist activates a certain percentage of the detector array so that information is acquired from a circular portion of the anatomic section. Built in to the SFOV selection are additional correction factors used to process different types of tissue. For example, a CT scanner may have a specific selection for scans of the head that attempt to limit the artifact that occurs at the delineation of bone and brain tissue. (Berland, 1987, p.45)
138. (c) The width of a window determines the range of pixel values that are assigned a shade of gray around a given level. In this example, all pixels within the range of −300 to +700 Hounsfield units will be assigned shades of gray. Pixels of less than −300 Hounsfield units will appear black, whereas pixels of more than +700 Hounsfield units will appear white. This calculation is performed by dividing the width in half and subtracting and adding this value to the level. (Berland, 1987, p.123)
139. (a) The section width of a CT image controls the length of the voxel. The dimensions of a voxel may also be reduced through decreases in the size of the pixel. Increases in matrix size and decreases in DFOV decrease the dimensions of the pixel and voxel. (Seeram, 1994, p.79)
140. (d) A CT image of a homogeneous material should have pixels with the same CT number. Any variation in CT number between pixels

indicates that noise has entered the system, causing a loss in accuracy. (Seeram, 1994, p.209)

141. (d) The first- and second-generation CT scanners used a translate–rotate method of data acquisition. The x-ray tube and detectors translated across the patient's head, recording transmission measurements. The entire system then rotated a certain number of degrees. This process of translation–rotation was repeated for 180°. First- and second-generation CT scanners used from 2–30 detectors. (Seeram, 1994, p.88)

142. (a) The transmitted intensity of a CT x-ray beam and the attenuation of the tissue imaged are inversely related. As the tissue begins to attenuate less radiation, the transmitted intensity of the beam increases. Areas of less dense tissue allow more radiation to pass onto the detectors, and vice versa. (Seeram, 1994 p.70)

143. (b) Because of its solid nature, the scintillation detector interacts with a higher percentage of incident x-ray photons, giving it a better capture, or intrinsic, efficiency. (Seeram, 1994, p.98)

144. (b) The third-generation CT scanner uses a fan beam projected onto a wide detector array. The third-generation CT x-ray beam is commonly mistaken for the "pencil beam" used with only two detectors in the first-generation CT scanner. (Seeram, 1994, p.89)

145. (a) The resolution test pattern embedded within this type of phantom is used to measure the spatial resolution of the CT scanner. The effects of different technical factors on spatial resolution may be examined by calculating the maximum number of visible line pairs. (Seeram, 1994, p.206)

146. (a) Pixels that differ by only 1 Hounsfield unit represent tissue whose attenuation coefficients differ by only 0.1%. (Wolbarst, 1993, p.321)

147. (b) Collimators reduce the intensity of the CT x-ray beam by absorbing the periphery of the beam. As they restrict the field size, the collimators absorb a portion of the radiation, thus reducing the beam intensity. A decrease in collimation increases the intensity of the x-ray beam. (Berland, 1987, p.23)

148. (c) Scintillation crystals are used in cooperation with photodiodes in a scintillation-type CT detector. The photodiode is a solid-state device that absorbs the light flashes given off by the crystal. The photodiode then emits an electrical signal in response to this light. (Seeram, 1994, p.99)

149. (b) The width of a CT window controls the range of pixel values that are assigned a shade of gray. The width is centered around a level that is equal to the value of the tissue of interest. (Berland, 1987, p.123)

150. (c) Spiral and helical CT scanners are a recent development in CT technology. The advent of slip-ring technology and improvements in x-ray tube design have made this innovation possible. Slip-rings have

taken the place of the cumbersome cables previously used to transmit the CT signal and supply power to the tube and detectors. This enables the tube and detectors to continuously rotate around the patient, acquiring data in the form of a helix. The longer exposure times of up to 60 seconds require extremely efficient x-ray tubes with enormous heat capacities. (Bushberg et al., 1994, p.259)

APPENDIX

Bibliography

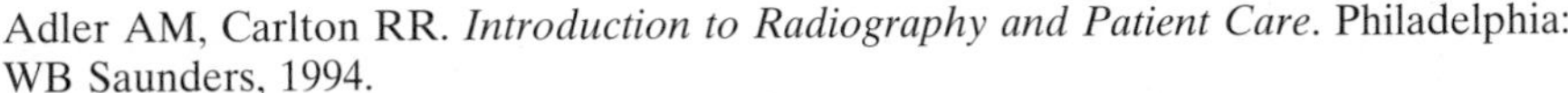

Adler AM, Carlton RR. *Introduction to Radiography and Patient Care*. Philadelphia: WB Saunders, 1994.

Ballinger PW. *Merrill's Atlas of Radiographic Positions and Radiologic Procedures*, 8th ed. St Louis: Mosby, 1995.

Barrett C, Anderson L, Holder L, Poliakoff S. *Primer of Sectional Anatomy with MRI and CT Correlation*, 2nd ed. Baltimore: Williams & Wilkins, 1994.

Berland LL. *Practical CT Technology and Techniques*. New York: Raven Press, 1987.

Bo W, Wolfman N, Krueger W, Meschan I. *Basic Atlas of Sectional Anatomy with Correlated Imaging*, 2nd ed. Baltimore: Williams & Wilkins, 1990.

Bushberg J, Seibert J, Leidholdt E, Boone J. *The Essential Physics of Medical Imaging*. Baltimore: Williams & Wilkins, 1994.

Carr DH. *Contrast Media*. London: Churchill Livingstone, 1988.

Chiu L, Lipcamon J, Yiu-Chiu V. *Clinical Computed Tomography for the Technologist*. New York: Raven Press, 1995.

Clemente CD. *Gray's Anatomy*, 13th ed. Philadelphia: Lea & Febiger, 1985.

Copstead LC. *Perspectives on Pathophysiology*. Philadelphia: WB Saunders, 1995.

Curry T, Dowdey J, Murry R. *Christensen's Physics of Diagnostic Radiology*, 4th ed. Philadelphia: Lea & Febiger, 1990.

Ehrlich RA, McCloskey ED. *Patient Care in Radiography*, 3rd ed. St Louis: Mosby, 1989.

Firooznia H, Golimbu C, Rafii M, Rauschning W, Weinreb J. *MRI and CT of the Musculoskeletal System*. St Louis: Mosby, 1992.

Fishman EK, Brooke JR Jr. *Spiral CT: Principles, Techniques and Clinical Applications*. New York: Raven Press, 1995.

Gedgaudas-McClees RK, Torres WE. *Essentials of Body Computed Tomography*. Philadelphia: WB Saunders, 1990.

Guyton AC. *Textbook of Medical Physiology*. Philadelphia: WB Saunders, 1986.

Katzberg RW. *The Contrast Media Manual*. Baltimore: Williams & Wilkins, 1992.

Lane A, Sharfaei H. *Modern Sectional Anatomy*. Philadelphia: WB Saunders, 1992.

Laudicina P, Wean D. *Applied Angiography for Radiographers*. Philadelphia: WB Saunders, 1994.

Lee J, Sagel S, Stanley R. *Computed Body Tomography with MRI Correlation*, 2nd ed. New York: Raven Press, 1989.

The Merck Manual, 15th ed. Rahway, NJ: Merck Sharp & Dohme Research Laboratories, 1987.

Mosby's Medical Dictionary, 4th ed. St Louis: Mosby, 1994.

Moss A, Gamsu G, Genant H. *Computed Tomography of the Body with Magnetic Resonance Imaging*, 2nd ed. Philadelphia, WB Saunders, 1992.

Putman C, Ravin C. *Textbook of Diagnostic Imaging*, 2nd ed. Philadelphia: WB Saunders, 1994.

Seeram E. *Computed Tomography*. Philadelphia: WB Saunders, 1994.

Snopek A. *Fundamentals of Special Radiographic Procedures*, 3rd ed. Philadelphia: WB Saunders, 1992.

Torres LS. *Basic Medical Techniques and Patient Care*, 4th ed. Philadelphia: JB Lippincott, 1993.

Tortorici MR, Apfel PJ. *Advanced Radiographic and Angiographic Procedures*. Philadelphia: FA Davis, 1995.

Wicke L. *Atlas of Radiologic Anatomy*, 5th ed (English). Philadelphia: Lea & Febiger, 1994.

Wolbarst AB. *Physics of Radiology*. Norwalk, CT: Appleton & Lange, 1993.